# PANDEMIC PERSPECTIVES

*A filmmaker's journey in 10 essays*

Howard Burton

Open Agenda Publishing

Copyright © Howard Burton 2022

First published in 2022 by Open Agenda Publishing Inc.
All rights reserved.

ISBN: 978-1-77170-302-4 (paperback)
ISBN: 978-1-77170-303-1 (hardcover)
ISBN: 978-1-77170-301-7 (ebook)
ISBN: 978-1-77170-305-5 (ePDF)
ISBN: 978-1-77170-304-8 (audiobook)

Visit www.ideasroadshow.com for details about the film, *Pandemic Perspectives*, and the series of podcasts with many of the film's participants.

# About the Author

Howard Burton is the author of four other books:

1. *Exceptionally Upsetting: How Americans are increasingly confusing knowledge with opinion & what can be done about it*
2. *Burning Down UNESCO: A Guide to Innovative Fundraising*
3. *Letters From Languedoc*
4. *First Principles: Building Perimeter Institute*

Visit www.howardburton.com for more details.

In 2012 he founded Ideas Roadshow, creating over 1000 videos and 120 books based upon detailed, long-format conversations with internationally renowned experts in a wide variety of different subject areas. Visit www.ideasroadshow.com for more details.

He holds a PhD in physics, an MA in philosophy, and was the founding executive director of Perimeter Institute for Theoretical Physics from 1999-2007. He lives in France.

# Acknowledgments

I would like to express my sincere gratitude to all 32 people involved in the *Pandemic Perspectives* film, many of whom were also forced to take a crash course in home cinematography and were remarkably good sports about the whole business.

Additional special thanks go to Noah and Louis Gershon for their heroic filming efforts while omicron was raging throughout the UK, Carl Castro for so promptly going to New Haven and almost going to Princeton, and Susan Wolf, whom I unfortunately couldn't convince to participate (as expected), but who quietly made an enormous contribution by connecting me to both Lorraine Daston and Paul Kahn.

As always, my wife Irena has been an emphatic rock of support; no words can possibly convey how much I am indebted to her superhuman combination of encouragement and understanding.

Lastly, I would like to thank Rhonda Brouwt at Open Agenda Publishing for her supreme editorial skills that somehow managed to convert my largely unintelligible meanderings into at least somewhat coherent prose. Suffice it to say that any lingering errors that the reader might encounter are my sole responsibility and have nothing to do with her.

*To the memory of Lewis Thomas (1913-1993)*

# Contents

1. In Search of Lewis Thomas ........................ 10
2. Reframing Education ................................ 25
3. Appreciating Science ................................ 48
4. Making Decisions ..................................... 59
5. Information & Misinformation ................. 78
6. Research, Evolving .................................... 96
7. Necessarily Global .................................. 116
8. Values ..................................................... 129
9. Biology, Better ........................................ 143
10. Conclusion ............................................ 168

# PANDEMIC PERSPECTIVES

*A filmmaker's journey in 10 essays*

# 1. In Search of Lewis Thomas

> "The record of the past half century has established, I think, two general principles about human disease. First, it is necessary to know a great deal about underlying mechanisms before one can really act effectively. Second, for every disease there is a single key mechanism that dominates all others."[1]

When the seriousness of the COVID-19 pandemic began to really sink in—when it could no longer be denied that, unlike SARS or MERS or any of the other potentially transformative global crises that had grabbed the headlines for a few days before simply fading away, this one was going to be different—the first thing I did was to head to my bookshelves to search for a copy of one of Lewis Thomas' books.

At the time, I was hardly what you might call a "Lewis Thomas fan." I owned two of his books—*The Medusa and the Snail* and *Late Night Thoughts on Listening to Mahler's Ninth Symphony*—both of which I vaguely remembered having leisurely thumbed through in the late 1990s, some 20 years or so after they'd been written.

But this time was different: No longer idly searching for a stimulating read to spice up my evening, now I needed help; and my lingering recollection was that, as increasingly panicked media reports of contagion moved from Wuhan to Bergamo to New York, Thomas' unique combination of lucid, penetrating writing skills and detailed biological understanding would be just the ticket.

---

[1] "Medical Lessons from History," in *The Medusa and the Snail*

Of course, I thought, since the books were written more than 40 years ago, it was inevitable that much would be out of date. But then, given that I knew next to nothing about biomedical matters and Thomas had been a hugely accomplished and wide-ranging physician, researcher and administrator, it seemed an appropriate place to start. Which it most certainly was. But what I hadn't bargained for was that the more I read, the manifestly less "out of date" it seemed.

I plunged in, naturally enough, with the essay "On Disease," mid-way through *The Medusa and the Snail*—eight and a half pages of penetrating prose, punctuated with regular invocations of technical terms that I immediately glossed over: lymphocytes, endotoxins, phagocytosis and so forth.

What I was searching for had nothing to do with official immunological jargon: I needed a reference point for our contemporary understanding of the nature of disease, an intellectual framework for comprehending what the hell was happening around me.

In fact, that's probably not right. More likely, what I was really looking for was confirmation of what I already "knew": that we live in a hostile world of zillions of microbial pathogens bent on destroying us, and the reason we manage to compete in this deadly zero-sum game of survival is thanks to our wonderfully sophisticated immune system honed by billions of years of evolution that can, in most cases anyway, manage to eventually destroy almost anything that nature throws at us.

But that's not what I got.

"On Disease" begins by talking of meningitis.

> *"The meningococcus, viewed from a distance, seems to have the characteristics of an implacable, dangerous enemy of the whole human race…But it is not so."*

It turns out, Thomas tells us, that of all the people infected with the bacteria in question, only a very small percentage go on to develop the terrible invasion of the central nervous system that is meningitis.

> *"The rule for meningococcal infection is a benign, transient infection of the upper respiratory tract, hardly an infection at all, more like an equable association."*

Why, then, does meningitis occur?

> *"It is still a mystery that meningitis develops in some patients, but it is unlikely that this represents a special predilection of the bacteria; it may be that the defense mechanisms of affected patients are flawed in some special way, so that the meningococci are granted access, invited in, so to say."*

From there we are taken on a rapid survey of a number of well-studied instances, from the generalized Shwartzman reaction to endotoxin shock, where the principal existential threat to an organism is not so much from the unrelenting determination of an invading pathogen but rather the host's own immune response—or, perhaps better put, "over-response"—to it.

This was not at all what I had expected. But it did, eerily, resonate strongly with an obvious question that increasingly surfaced as the COVID-19 storm rapidly swept over us and hospital staff began to speak of the fatal impact of "cytokine storms": Why were some people dying from being infected with a virus that others didn't even notice they had?

It resonated, too, with something vastly more mundane that had long perplexed me: Why, exactly, do I have to ice a sprained ankle? I've played enough sports to know that whenever a minor injury occurs, the standard treatment for the first few days is "RICE"—rest, ice, compression and elevation—to "treat the inflammation and reduce the swelling." Which definitely works. But why? Why on earth should it make sense to be officiously interfering with my body's spontaneous reaction to a routine injury that was presumably honed by billions of years of evolution? What's going on? Should tigers out in the savanna be properly icing *their* sprained ankles in order to more successfully dominate their habitat?

Of course I was aware that there were people who were known to have specific issues with their immune system—the so-called "immunocompromised" or "immunodeficient"—and thus had the misfortune to often suffer deeply from a range of afflictions that the rest of us could fight off with relative ease, just as those who had problems with their lungs or heart were more susceptible to pneumonia or coronary disease, but that's clearly a different sort of situation.

Most people, I had naturally assumed, were blessed with immune systems that worked optimally in order to fend off the constant onslaught of invading pathogens. But that seems to be a decidedly naive way of looking at it. And once you stop regarding the immune system as a perfectly-tuned machine and more like a work in progress— staggeringly effective most of the time and in most cases, but a work in progress nonetheless—the picture becomes vastly more nuanced.

So that was the first big shock.

The second shock was that the timeworn image of us engaged in a perpetual battle with a pathogen-infested world out to destroy us at every turn is, well, flat-out wrong.

Of course, there are lots of nasty things out there and our immune systems are mind-bogglingly wondrous at being able to protect us from them in all sorts of remarkably comprehensive ways, but while Thomas unhesitatingly avers that modern advances in sanitation, nutrition and housing have correspondingly transformed public health by dramatically reducing the risk of infection from such would-be attackers, he consistently takes aim at the popular perception that we are locked in an unremitting Darwinian duel with the microbial world.

> *"It is true, of course, that germs are all around us; they comprise a fair proportion of the sheer bulk of the soil, and they abound in the air. But it is certainly not true that they are our natural enemies. Indeed, it comes as a surprise to realize that such a tiny minority of the bacterial populations of the earth has any interest at all in us. The commonest of encounters between bacteria and the higher forms of life take place after the death of the latter, in the course of recycling the elements of life. This is obviously the main business of the microbial world in general, and it has nothing to do with disease."*

Moreover—and it is a very big moreover—it's not just that most of the microbial world ignores us, it is that, in a very real way, we are actually *dependent* on them. Opinions vary these days about the exact ratio between microbial cells and human cells in the average human body—a decade or so ago it was thought to be 10:1 and present estimates are about 1:1—but given that we are talking about some $10^{13}$ human cells, an order of magnitude or two hardly makes any difference in getting the point across. The prospect of having roughly 30 000 000 000 000 microbes inside each and every one of our bodies, many of which are actively engaged in a symbiotic relationship with us so as to directly help us perform a range of essential human functions, gives a strikingly different picture to the "us vs them/zap the invader" framework we are constantly bombarded with.

And lest you be thinking, *Well, perhaps that's the case for bacteria, but what about viruses?* It turns out not to matter one jot. Indeed, in a later essay,[2] Thomas speculates on a possible key evolutionary role that viruses might play in *"picking up odds and ends of DNA from their*

---
[2] "The Art and Craft of Memoir" in *The Fragile Species*

*hosts and then passing these around, as though at a great party,"* given that, *"After all, we live in a sea of our own viruses, most of which seem to be there for no purpose, not even to make us sick."*

He continues musingly:

> *"We can hope that some of them might be taking hold of useful items of genetic news from time to time, then passing these along for the future of the race. It makes a cheerful footnote, anyway: next time you feel a cold coming on, reflect on the possibility that you may be giving a small boost to evolution."*

At this point it might be worth stepping back and taking a moment to emphasize that I am most definitely not some kind of perversely virusphilic fellow who greeted the arrival of the COVID-19 pandemic with a cheerful Panglossian shrug, wistfully wondering what sort of potential, long-term evolutionary benefit *Homo sapiens* might receive in exchange for us being locked in our homes for a while. Like everyone else, I am most emphatically committed to doing whatever it takes to somehow rid the world of SARS-CoV-2, or at least render it as benign as possible to my fellow humans.

But in order to appreciate how best to do that, it seemed obviously imperative to have a genuine understanding of the very basics of what is actually going on in the biological world around me; and the more I read, the more astounded I became to discover that, in fact, I had no real clue.

In particular, if the dominant world-view that had been significantly reinforced by the onset of the pandemic—that we are single-mindedly locked in a 24/7 kill-or-be-killed war with our hostile environment—is actually a considerably distorted picture of reality, it would be best to remedy that as quickly as possible before I find myself irretrievably alienated from my surroundings. It was bad enough that I'd suddenly found myself instinctively crossing the street whenever I'd glimpse others casually ambling towards me (especially children!) and washing my hands at every conceivable opportunity.

So, what to do?

Well, read more, for starters. Not only all the works of Lewis Thomas, but also the many online resources that were freely available at the click of a mouse, from the CDC to the Institut Pasteur to a plethora of comprehensive review articles on PubMed. And then there were videos—often a much more efficient way of quickly getting a handle on the required basics for a neophyte such as myself. A staple of mine in those early days was the highly informative and pedagogically sound *Zero to Finals* series, which had the added bonus of strongly appealing to my sense of irony that I, of all people, would one day find myself diligently poring over material created for medical students.

As part of my on-again, off-again dance with "the real world," my largely misspent youth was filled with professional forays and half-forays in just about every conceivable direction as I meandered through various degrees in physics and philosophy. I took the GMAT and LSAT, almost applied to law school, almost began an MBA program, almost worked on Wall St, and almost did a large number of other things besides. Virtually the only career path I never even remotely contemplated for one moment was that of a physician—medicine being a topic where success was obviously predicated upon the rote memorization of specific stages of repulsiveness in obscure Latin nomenclature. Yet here I was, decades later, repeatedly watching Tom Watchman's *Understanding the Immune System in One Video* like someone cramming for his immunology finals. There's nothing, it seems, that a global pandemic cannot do.

Meanwhile, in addition to independently reading books and trawling the internet, another obvious way forward was to try to concoct a way to combine my newfound biological interest with my current professional life.

Back in 2012, I started a digital media initiative called Ideas Roadshow that was dedicated to capturing accessible expert insights in various formats for a non-specialist audience. Why not make a film about key biological issues for the general public, spurred on by the global pandemic and "leveraging" my transparently obvious position of puzzled biological ignoramus? Surely there would be lots of people interested in watching that sort of thing at the moment?

Obviously, given the circumstances, normal on-site filming wasn't going to be possible, but as the world had rapidly shifted to interacting via Zoom and the like, it seemed feasible to contemplate doing things remotely, particularly as most experts I would be involving were affiliated to academic or research institutions that had ready access to studios and filming facilities.

Filled with enthusiasm, I set off looking for suitable experts to talk to. Based on my past experiences, there must be hundreds, if not thousands, of engaging, internationally-acknowledged experts anxious to harness this moment to publicly ruminate on wider issues, from current conceptual misunderstandings to a litany of pressing open questions in immunology, virology, epidemiology and more.

The only issue, it seemed, was that, given the sheer breadth of relevant topics and the consequent volume of specialists around the globe, there were simply too many people to choose from. Well, I told myself, that's a good problem to have—just dive in and see what happens.

So I did. And what occurred was so remarkable that I still can't hardly believe it: almost nobody agreed to participate. Every day I would send off roughly a hundred investigatory emails to biomedical researchers all over the world. And of those hundred, I'd typically get about ten or so replies, politely (or sometimes not so politely) demurring, with the other 90% never bothering to respond at all.

I was flabbergasted. Over years of cold-calling people for Ideas Roadshow, I typically heard back from about 90%, with about 60% of those eventually agreeing to participate in whatever I was proposing. And now, when the whole world was suddenly clamoring for meaningful biomedical guidance, my response rate had plummeted roughly three orders of magnitude, to somewhere between 0.1% and 0.2%.

What was going on?

It couldn't be a "reputation issue." While Ideas Roadshow is hardly a household name, there was clearly much that had been done to convince anyone who bothered looking that it was a genuine endeavor that many serious people had been involved in. At this point I had held long-format conversations with well over 100 acknowledged specialists in political theory, physics, history, linguistics, neuroscience, philosophy and more, many of whom held very strong international reputations and positions at some of the world's most famous institutions. It might not be your thing, but it was clearly *a* thing, of sorts.

Well, you might be tempted to argue, in the midst of a constantly-shifting global pandemic experts with specialized biomedical skills were far too busy to engage in anything outside of the laboratory, but then all too often I would see the very same people I contacted appear on CNN or BBC or as authors of op-eds for major newspapers. And however busy immunologists and epidemiologists might be—and they certainly were of course—it was universally acknowledged that in these times of crisis it was essential to provide members of the general public with reliable, accessible information—which was precisely the sort of activity that I was trying to do.

After a time I concluded that the problem didn't have much to do with me or Ideas Roadshow or reputation or any of that—it had to do with my approach, what I was asking them to participate in.

Because unlike the other "media and outreach responsibilities" they were often engaged in, I wasn't interested in them simply holding forth on what policymakers should do or detail how a virus might spread throughout the population or enter a cell, but was rather requesting that they involve themselves in a broad-based discussion with me on what it all means, harnessing the dynamic of conversation between myself, a curious non-specialist, and them as experts.

The point, of course, isn't for me to pretend that I am on their level, or to presume that I can somehow "collaborate" with them to address outstanding questions in the field, but to simply harness the opportunity of talking to someone who knows in order to get a much deeper sense of what is actually going on than we're typically presented with through the usual channels. This is what I've been doing for the better part of a decade, whether it's grappling with the subtleties of ancient Aegean scripts or trying to get a handle on the neurological mechanisms of human memory.

It's hardly a novel approach: anyone who's given a public talk on her research—which is pretty well everyone these days—is familiar with the basic idiom. The only difference here is that this isn't a talk, but a conversation between themselves and a keen layperson anxious to forthrightly deepen his understanding of what the current research landscape looks like: what we know, what we don't and why.

Lewis Thomas, I'm convinced, would surely have understood. Most unfortunately, however, he was no longer available, having died in 1993. And it was hard to escape the conclusion that most of his intellectual descendants seemed far more interested in harnessing the moment to make pronouncements than engage in anything like an open discussion of wider-ranging issues.

The final nail in my putative "A Physicist Tries to Understand Biology" film occurred after a remote conversation with one of the few specialists who *did* agree to engage: a highly-accomplished scientist whose major focus these days is on trying to develop vaccines through the implementation of so-called "broadly neutralizing antibodies."

The very notion of a "broadly neutralizing antibody" was immediately captivating to me, and seemed to naturally open up all sorts of possible avenues to a detailed understanding of fundamental processes of the immune system.

The standard picture, as I understand it, is that most of the time contact with a specific pathogen results in the immune system eventually producing particular antibodies that are finely "tuned" to neutralizing that specific pathogen, but that in some instances there exist antibodies that somehow have the capacity of neutralizing a somewhat wider set of such pathogens, and are hence "broadly neutralizing" in this context.

Given that a major challenge of neutralizing a virus is that it has an annoying tendency to keep evolving and thus evading, or at least diminishing, the effectiveness of whatever specific neutralizing element the body throws at it—something that is obviously uppermost on everyone's minds these days—the notion that it might be possible to somehow come up with a class of antibodies that has the capacity to incapacitate a broad evolutionary range of viruses is obviously a potential game-changer.

Equally importantly, it seemed to me, it could shed light on all sorts of vital mechanistic details that we might not yet fully grasp: How, exactly, do antibodies neutralize pathogens anyway? What, precisely, are the different approaches and what do they depend on? Why are some more successful in some circumstances than others?

The more I thought about it, the more excited I became; and, as tends to happen, the more questions popped into my head: To what extent could you rigorously characterize the notion of what it means to be a "broadly neutralizing antibody"? Are all antibodies potentially "broadly neutralizing" if looked at in the right way? If not, why not? Might it be possible to imagine a sort of mathematical space of all types of antibodies with smaller subspaces representing "broadly neutralizing antibodies"? If so, what do those subspaces depend on?

At its heart, this whole question of "broadly neutralizing antibodies" struck me as a potentially transformative window on how we might meaningfully categorize the range of possible evolutionary trajectories of a pathogen, together with, of course, our efforts to combat it: for at some point, depending on how you set things up, the virus could presumably evolve out of the range of where such a "broadly neutralizing antibody" could neutralize it and then you'd have some sense of where the boundaries are, as it were, and what that might mean—which would be huge. Or maybe for some types of pathogens there are actually no such boundaries and it is somehow constrained to evolve within a space where it would always be susceptible to the broadly neutralizing antibody, which might be huger still.

Or maybe somehow all of this is nonsense (this often happens when I get excited) and I have assumed something obviously wrong somewhere that my interlocutor can promptly straighten me out about.

The way I figured it I couldn't lose, so I was extremely looking forward to the chance to discuss the implications associated with these deeply curious broadly neutralizing antibodies with him in detail.

Unfortunately, it never happened. That is, the discussion technically occurred, but frustratingly enough, it somehow never went anywhere near any of the core issues, as we kept talking straight past each other.

So far as I could tell, his attitude was something along the lines of, "*A broadly neutralizing antibody is something that you find in a lab which neutralizes different variants of a pathogen and that's all there is to it, so put away all your fancy-pants talk of mathematical subspaces,*" with the corresponding implication that I was desperately trying to somehow show him up, or show off, or be a "physics imperialist," or whatever.

It wasn't just a disagreement about ideas—in fact, it wasn't a disagreement about ideas at all, given that it was patently obviously that I had no ideas. I just had questions. But somehow, bizarrely, all of my questions were interpreted as a personal affront. Maybe this was why, I mused to myself, so many biomedical researchers had been unwilling to talk to me. They didn't want to answer my questions. They didn't even want to *listen* to my questions. They just wanted to make pronouncements.

We had come, very depressingly, very far indeed from Dr Thomas' determination to joyfully speculate on future scientific possibilities.

In time, I did manage to find some enthusiastic biomedical experts to involve in my effort: the Chief of Research at Toronto's Hospital for Sick Children who was a leading force in the co-discovery of genetic copy number variation; a Brazilian neuroscientist who found himself trapped in São Paulo when the pandemic broke out and returned to his epidemiological roots to assist the country in its time of need; an evolutionary biologist who's an expert on "fitness landscapes" (and who unhesitatingly assures me that such a picture is the obviously appropriate way to interpret my intuitive notion of "mathematical subspaces" mentioned earlier) and a young postdoctoral researcher at Stanford who developed an intriguing model of viral mutations using a machine-learning technique for natural language processing (something I'm certain the linguistically and etymologically-obsessed Lewis Thomas would have found completely captivating). I even eventually located a thoughtful and decidedly non-hubristic immunologist who has recently written an engaging and accessible popular book on the basics of how the body fends off infectious diseases.[3]

But even more significantly, it gradually began to dawn on me that, for all the opportunities the pandemic presented for deepening our biological understanding, it afforded even more meaningful occasions to uniquely examine a number of vital sociological issues, from public policy to contemporary social values.

In retrospect, it's clear to me that, given the wide range of pressing societal issues that have been profoundly illuminated by the pandemic, I should have started off this way from the outset. However fascinating the intricacies of viral-host mechanisms might be, the need to critically

---

[3] *Infectious* by John Tregoning

examine to what extent the current crisis reveals essential gaps in our social fabric is obviously considerably more pressing.

The film, then, naturally broadened in focus. And as it gained momentum, I eventually decided to broaden things still further by turning the documentary itself into one component of a larger project that includes 24 detailed podcast conversations and this book.

This way, I figured, people would be offered a trio of overlapping options: a film showcasing a range of brief expert insights, more detailed individual reflections through the conversational medium of podcasts and this book of a "behind the scenes" perspective to supply some overarching context, together with my own evolving views.

And evolve they most certainly did. But through it all, one factor remained intriguingly constant: no matter where my investigations led—reforming our educational priorities, balancing basic and applied research, contrasting medicine and biomedical research, investigating the decision-making process, confronting our moral obligations to the less fortunate—I was struck by the fact that Lewis Thomas had already been there, writing eloquently and penetratingly about them well over 40 years ago, as the introductory quotations of each chapter so vividly attest to.

It is not so much that we don't know these things, or have nobody to point us in the right direction, or even need a global pandemic to jolt us into re-appraising matters, it is that we have an unfortunate tendency to steadfastly ignore those perspicacious few who have gone to great lengths to alert us of their fundamental importance.

Lewis Thomas, an extraordinarily compassionate and fertile writer who was as deeply embedded in the scientific establishment of his day as could possibly be imagined, clearly did not manage, for all his literary and professional success, to engender a legacy of successive generations of similarly thoughtful, humble and unabashedly curious biomedical researchers. That is, of course, hardly his fault. But it is certainly a profound shame, and one well worth drawing attention to. We need his like now more than ever.

As I write these words, growing numbers of people appear to be convinced that the pandemic is, if not completely over, at least thankfully moving towards a different stage, allowing us to finally begin returning to something like our previous prepandemic lives. Should that come to pass—and I desperately hope that it will, although it would certainly be wise not to be rashly optimistic given everything we've seen over the past couple of years—there will naturally be a significant temptation to put all that's happened behind us and forget everything about the last two years as quickly as possible.

But that, I'm convinced, would be a big mistake. The COVID-19 pandemic was—indeed, still is—horribly destructive, profoundly disturbing and overwhelmingly exhausting. Let's at least try to learn something from it.

# 2. Reframing Education

> *"The worst thing that has happened to science education is that the great fun has gone out of it. Very few see science as the high adventure it really is, the wildest of all explorations ever undertaken by human beings. Instead they become baffled early on, and they are misled into thinking that bafflement is simply the result of not having learned all the facts. They are not told, as they should be told, that everyone else is baffled as well."*[1]

Education has to be the strangest area in all of public policy. Virtually everyone agrees that it is one of the most essential things to be doing well, yet almost nobody agrees on what "doing well" actually means. Worse, there is precious little coherent movement towards the development of any clearly defined ways of practically assessing what "success" might actually look like. And infinitely worse still, there is a constant, gnawing lack of awareness—indeed, even acknowledgment—of these fundamental impediments to any genuine move towards progress. It's hard to envision how we might in any meaningful way "improve our educational systems" if we are completely in the dark about where we should be going, let alone how to do so.

Of course it is complicated. Very complicated even. But that's all the more reason, one might think, for rolling up our sleeves and trying to puzzle out at least how to begin.

Part of the complication, I think, is that "the education system" is a large, sprawling, multi-headed beast that incorporates a vast number

---

1   "Humanities and Science" in *Late Night Thoughts on Listening to Mahler's Ninth Symphony*

of key societal concerns, from finding the best preschool to getting the most out of college to learning essential job-retraining skills. Given this exceptionally broad landscape, it's hardly surprising that our intuitive sense of the corresponding goals in play varies enormously. Most would agree, for example, that the fundamental mission of a preschool is to provide broad-based stimulation and generate a love of learning rather than instill dollops of subject-specific knowledge, while the proper role of college, say, is tilted in precisely the other direction.

Most, but not all. For that, too, is part of the confusion. Proponents of a general liberal arts curriculum will unhesitatingly hold forth on the intrinsic merits of personal development and human flourishing, thereby loudly butting heads with those who insist that all of those hand-waving lofty sentiments are merely an indulgent distraction from the core business of post-secondary education, which is to prepare young people for the workforce.

And such divisions get obscured almost beyond recognition when general education advocates respond, as they increasingly do, with the suspiciously tactical claim that, along with nourishing one's soul, a liberal arts education also turns out to have the added bonus of giving students a significant competitive advantage in a complex and rapidly-changing job market.

Into this turbulent muddle strode the COVID-19 pandemic, summarily closing classrooms around the globe and abruptly ushering in the age of "enforced online learning."

This was, to say the very least, unsettling. But given the profound incoherence that had long beset the world of educational policy, I couldn't help but wonder if it didn't also represent an opportunity of sorts. Physicists often like to invoke "thought experiments" to push an idea to its logical limits in order to see where it might break down or what hitherto unforeseen implications of the theoretical framework might be revealed. Imagine a world without electromagnetism, say, or a universe with just one particle in it. What would happen? What would it look like?

It's a wonderful trick, and often yields startlingly acute insights that you wouldn't otherwise notice, illuminating vital dependencies or independencies that had been long masked by standard assumptions associated with our usual world view that we had unreflectively endorsed.

For some reason such approaches don't seem to have ever caught on in the social sciences, but suddenly we found ourselves in the completely unimaginable scenario where a fiendish sociological thought experiment, *Imagine a world where all standard educational practices would suddenly be shut down*, actually happened. It was deeply disturbing of course, and hardly the sort of thing one would ever seriously consider doing in the normal course. But now that it *had* occurred, it only seemed reasonable to try to take some sort of advantage of it. Surely other people had similar thoughts?

Well, not so much, it seemed. As far as I could tell, virtually everyone looked to be focused on how to navigate the tools of online education we were suddenly stuck with to simulate, as best as possible, the standard personal, face to face, type of classroom experience that we were all used to.

Meanwhile, as the crisis dragged on, alarmist voices began summarily declaring that the pandemic had produced a debilitating "education gap" that would irreparably damage the prospects of those trapped in "the COVID generation," once more demonstrating the ability of "educational experts" to capriciously transcend the tiresome constraints of evidence-based investigations whenever it suited.

I did stumble upon one educational theorist, however, who took a rather different approach. In his beguilingly-named article, "Tofu is Not Cheese: Rethinking Education Amid the COVID-19 Pandemic,"

Yong Zhao provocatively wrote: "*This is a crisis, but within which is the opportunity to rethink education.*"

Yong, an education professor at the University of Kansas and Melbourne Graduate School of Education, urged us to go beyond trying to "*pretend we can make online education the same as face-to-face schools*" (analogous to doggedly maintaining that tofu is cheese despite all the obvious evidence to the contrary, in case you were wondering where that fit in). He goes on to point out that the standard question aimed at online education: *Does it work?* is actually both meaningless and dangerous—meaningless, because the extent to which something can be regarded as "working" naturally depends on the corresponding outcomes you are measuring, and those are typically all over the map. But it is also dangerous, because focusing our attention on trying to somehow assess an undefinable level of "effectiveness" naturally wastes valuable resources and distracts us from vital questions that can and should be addressed, such as: *What, exactly, is worth teaching and learning?*

Yong's personal answer to that question revolves around what he calls (and, agreeably, actually defines) "global competency" and "digital competency," before tackling how we might go about implementing those changes in practice.

All in all it was a refreshingly different approach and one that resonated quite strongly with the sorts of things that I had been hoping that educational theorists would be thinking about. Individual solutions to the question of what should be done would naturally vary, but as long as the focus was on explicitly capitalizing on the unique, external shock to the system provided by the pandemic, there seemed serious cause for optimism.

Of course, just having theorists seriously contemplate how we might reimagine education from the ground up was hardly a guarantee that any transformative new developments would actually happen: there is often a yawning gap from theory to practice in any field, and none more so than when one is forced to coordinate between rigidly stratified levels of a deeply conservative bureaucracy; but at least it's a start, and one that the pandemic had given particular impetus to.

As Yong emphasized during our subsequent remote-filming session, the sudden cessation of "business as usual" practices caused by the pandemic has the potential to jolt us into a more heightened state of "big picture" awareness.

> *"This stop creates a space for teachers and students to imagine what education can be, because before we were always talking about how education cannot change because of the traditional conventions and practices."*

But then the question immediately poses itself: So? To what extent *have* we actually capitalized on this "space" we've been presented with? Sadly, not very much:

> *"I don't think that people have taken advantage of the opportunities created by the pandemic to rethink education. By and large schools are eager to return to normal to deliver education in the classroom as they did before. We have not got together to imagine what the future could be."*

But perhaps it was naive to look for all-encompassing signs of transformative change at such an early stage. Maybe a more productive approach would be to focus more narrowly on how the pandemic has illuminated the benefits of specific techniques and practices hitherto unappreciated. A good person to call on for help here, I thought to myself, was Stephen Kosslyn.

I first met Stephen about 7 years earlier when he was the Founding Dean of Minerva Schools, a new, private university in San Francisco launched by businessman Ben Nelson. The longtime Dean of Social Science at Harvard University, Stephen is an internationally-renowned cognitive psychologist who was one of the first in his field to capitalize on the potential of then-nascent brain-imaging technologies.

More recently, he has firmly established himself as a global leader in the science of learning, whose primary focus these days is on promoting the manifold benefits of "active learning."

While some refer to active learning as "learning by doing," Stephen prefers the more revealing "learning by using," pointing out that "doing" is an unhelpfully nebulous term which might well refer to almost anything. The whole point of active learning, he enthuses, is to achieve something concrete with some initially received information, directly demonstrating its relevance and utility by successfully applying it to the attainment of some specific goal.

Given that this can be achieved in many different ways and in many different circumstances, educators should constantly be on the lookout to invoke the particular approach that is most strongly fitted to the goals, strengths and constraints of the project at hand. Sometimes that involves doing things synchronously, with students and teachers engaged in simultaneous real-time activities, while other times it involves asynchronous interaction, such as independently pursuing various stages of a "flipped classroom." Revealingly too, sometimes the best setting is "in person" and sometimes it is "online." In other words, there is no one "ideal setting." It depends on the situation.

And one of the most striking early impacts of the pandemic, he pointed out, was that a good many educators who had never before seriously contemplated using online teaching suddenly discovered that they now had some active learning approaches that were considerably more effective than what they had been using in their normal face-to-face teaching.

In that sense, then, the pandemic definitely helped spark an increased recognition of pedagogical opportunities, dramatically revealing a spectrum of previously uncontemplated active learning options easily accessible through online techniques. Unfortunately, however, little of that had reached the popular consciousness, where a stark dichotomy between "online" and "normal" teaching has become steadily ingrained over time, with online teaching consistently viewed as, at best, a pale substitute for "the real classroom."

> *"I would have hoped that with all the parents looking over the shoulders of their children studying online that the parents would come to appreciate what educators were trying to do. But as far as I can tell, from reading and talking to various people, that hasn't happened very much. And I think part of the reason for that is that a lot of what goes on in education behind the scenes stays behind the scenes."*

Much as I was sympathetic to Stephen's determination to move beyond an inappropriate emphasis on the modes of teacher-student interaction and instead focus on assessing individual student learning outcomes, for me the single greatest educational question raised by the pandemic well and truly transcended any type of formal pedagogical setting: *To what extent could it be reasonably maintained that we actually live in a "well-educated society" at all?*

Like most people, I suppose, this is a topic I've occasionally pondered. I'm old enough to have heard various mutterings of an "educational crisis" in many places for decades, and have witnessed the birth, and death, of numerous government programs that were specifically designed to address it.[2]

In France, where I live, there is a regular cycle of "educational reform" every couple of years that begins with triumphant government declarations of long-overdue measures designed to dramatically improve the country's ability to harness its human capital and thereby enhance

---

[2] In the United States alone: *Goals 2000, No Child Left Behind, Race to the Top, Common Core*, and quite likely many more I'm forgetting.

its international competitiveness, followed by traffic-snarling protests from enraged educators loudly decrying the insidious abandonment of long-cherished republican principles before, inevitably, quietly petering out—which, come to think of it, neatly sums up many aspects of French public life.

Meanwhile, the OECD's PISA[3] has been comparing the mathematical, science and reading skills of 15-year-old students across many nations since 2000, the main effect of which seems to be a combination of chest-beating rhetoric from the winners and shoulder-shrugging affirmations of irrelevance from the losers.

The United States never seems to manage to crack the top 10 of any of the three PISA categories, and often is outside the top 20, but can nonetheless take solace in the fact that any objective ranking of global universities is overwhelmingly dominated by a litany of American institutions.

All in all it is pretty hard to take the whole business terribly seriously, which is why most of us didn't. But then along comes a global pandemic, and suddenly the streets are regularly filled with angry mobs insisting that a bevy of state-of-the art vaccines are the nefarious products of an evil government determined to poison you, and equally suddenly the question, *To what extent could it reasonably be maintained that we actually live in a well-educated society?* becomes thumpingly, overwhelmingly, relevant. Because I don't care how well you might have scored on your PISA test, or how many degrees you have from institutions at the very top of the Shanghai Rankings, if you are the slightest bit sensitive to the idea that you are in an appropriate position to opine on the specific merits of an antiviral vaccine when you've never made the effort to develop any clear understanding of what a virus actually **is**, then you most definitely ain't educated.

---

[3] Programme for International Student Assessment

Now it's important to be super-explicit here, because this is, I think, a key point. What I am most definitely *not* saying is that authority figures should be blindly trusted, or that one should never protest against government measures or that the only people who are qualified to make an informed assessment about how to proceed in a health crisis are those with a PhD in molecular biology. As it happens, I don't believe any of those things.

Instead what I'm driving at is the hugely important, and often dangerously overlooked, distinction between being educated and possessing knowledge. The two overlap, of course, but there are essential, subtle differences between them—differences that, to my mind anyway, are intimately tied to the question that began this chapter: How might we somehow "harness" the pandemic to better appreciate the true value of public education?

When discussing these sorts of things, the phrase "critical thinking" often comes to the fore, but on the whole I'm generally not a fan of that expression, not least because it strikes me as teetering precipitously close to a tautology—is there such a thing as "non-critical" thinking?—and tautologies are notoriously unhelpful things to invoke when you're trying to make any sort of intellectual progress. In short, it seems to me that all you've done by introducing the term "critical thinking" is simply tasked yourself with something else that you'll need to define at the outset; worse still, since it's an expression in common parlance, almost everybody out there has her own idea of what it means, so you'll be forced to expend considerable time and effort trying to convince people to abandon their own definitions for yours. What's the point?

Instead, let me start with a thought experiment. Let's imagine that we are somehow put in charge of singlehandedly transforming the entire education system—let's start with K–12, which is clearly the most significant, not to mention the hardest to change—and are forced to answer one simple question: *What are the five essential things that all students leaving high school should be in firm possession of in order to enable us to confidently declare that our educational system is "doing well"?*

Constraints have this wonderful ability to focus the mind; and the hope is that, by limiting ourselves to only five characteristics, a natural prioritization process will occur that might produce a measurable end-product, as opposed to vague, sanctimonious phrases like "critical thinking" that have a suspiciously smug, "all we're really aiming for is to put ourselves in a situation where everyone around us has the good sense to just act like we do" air about them. And by nebulously referring to the desired measurables as "things" that all students "should be in firm possession of," we're conspicuously avoiding any explicit invocations—for the moment anyway—of "knowledge," leaving the door open for a much wider interpretation.

Lastly, the criterion that **all** students should possess these requirements in order for the system as a whole to be deemed successful naturally reinforces the essential notion that any well-functioning educational system we develop must explicitly resonate with our core democratic principles. I will spare bombarding you with a litany of pithy quotes, from Jefferson to Dewey to Gandhi on how a well-functioning democracy is intrinsically dependent on the education of its citizenry (although they certainly exist), because the point is largely viewed as incontrovertible. Yet despite all of that, we in self-proclaimed democratic societies have nonetheless built our formative educational structures in such a way that it is widely accepted that they inevitably produce "winners and losers" and therefore should not be judged, or at least judged severely, by any consequent lack of comprehensiveness amongst all of the citizenry. The uneducated, it is assumed, like the poor, will always be with us.

This has long struck me as very strange.

If instead we adhered to the view that only a specialized elite should be in charge of governing the rest of us, then it would clearly make sense to have our educational structures focused on ensuring the appropriate intellectual development of those important few, since they were the ones who "mattered," as it were. Which is, naturally enough, exactly the sort of thing that Plato—no democrat he—famously detailed in his *Republic*.

But since we now explicitly take a very different approach, proclaiming that *all* the citizenry should play a fundamental role in how our key decisions are arrived at, then surely a vital function of our public education system is to equip the entire citizenry with the ability to constructively engage in these vital decision-making processes.

Of course it hardly follows that this is the *only* thing that our educational systems must do (obvious additional goals include the acquisition of a range of knowledge and skills to facilitate economic and social progress on both a societal and individual level), nor does it in any way imply that abandoning the prism of "winners and losers" means that we are forced to invoke some sort of vapid neo-Orwellian, pseudo-egalitarian, "everyone's a winner" rhetoric that in any way limits the notion of merit, ability or individual orientation.

All we are saying is that if a primary goal of our public educational system is to ensure that our societies are run as well as possible, and if the mechanisms for running our societies are manifestly dependent on **all** the citizenry, then the only coherent way to evaluate the degree of success or failure of such a system is to forthrightly consider to what extent it is having a beneficial impact on **everyone**.

But instead, as we nod our heads sagely at whatever insightful similar sentiments from Roosevelt or Mandela meander into our phones, we continue to regard public education primarily as a vehicle to enable meritorious individuals to attain success in the social hierarchy, while simultaneously disdaining the idea that our educational system should have some profound and long-lasting impact on the hearts and minds of everyday people as irredeemably elitist.

Ordinary citizens, it is clearly implied—indeed, often explicitly stated—don't need to endure any sort of externally imposed state-authorized "system" in order to learn how to make good decisions. They are born knowing how to do that; or at least their life experience, coupled with their innate common sense, is more than sufficient.

Well, you can't have it both ways. Either a public educational system is necessary for a democratic society to thrive or it isn't. You can argue that as currently constructed it is doing a good job or a bad job, but you can't coherently claim that the whole thing is both essential and irrelevant.

With these thoughts in mind, then, let's now return to the thought experiment at hand: What are the five essential things that all students leaving high school should be in firm possession of so that we can confidently declare that our educational system has sufficiently prepared citizens to productively engage in democratic decision-making?

Once again, I think that the pandemic has things to teach us here—well, it has certainly taught me, fortunate as I was to find myself catapulted into a situation where I had the chance to talk with so many thoughtful, experienced people who could help inform my judgment, coupled with the obligation to eventually produce something coherent from the whole business.

Here, then, is my answer to the question, my own personal "top five":

1. A strong command of basic mathematics and language skills

2. An appreciation of science

3. An awareness of the basic history of their country

4. A detailed understanding of how their government works

5. An ability to assess claims and evaluate evidence

Before diving into specific justifications and purported implications associated with this list, I think it's worth taking a moment to reiterate the fundamental goal of the exercise: to produce a list of five measurable characteristics that, should everyone possess them, would justify the claim that our education system is "successful" in terms of fulfilling its core mandate of developing citizens so as to best ensure the proper functioning of our democratic societies.

I am certainly not arguing that these are the only things that our educational systems should be doing, nor that this is the sum total of the things that all individuals, young or old, should be broadly encouraged to be engaged in. In particular, I'm most definitely not implying that it is a waste of time to become intimately familiar with Shakespeare or Confucianism or the intricacies of Formula One racing,[4] only that these are the essential goals to evaluate in order for us to be in a position of coherently evaluating to what extent our educational system is, or is not, "working well."

Rather more subtly, I'm also conspicuously silent on the specific details of the implied "evaluation process." What, precisely, would be involved, I can imagine someone asking, in determining to what extent a student has "a strong command" of basic mathematics? Well, I'm not going to answer that, largely because I don't pretend to actually know; but I'm very confident that there is a plethora of experienced educators out there who can proffer meaningful responses and eventually come to some sort of agreement on the matter. Put another way, if that is our principal stumbling block, then we're really in trouble.

Let me instead try to explain what I mean by each of the five areas and why I'm convinced that each must be included.

Fundamental mathematics and language skills are meta-requirements: giving people the necessary basics to do the other four. It is impossible to evaluate a statistical claim, for example, if you can't sufficiently parse

---

[4] This is probably true, actually

the words to appreciate what, exactly, is being claimed—or, for that matter, if you don't have any basic understanding of statistics. So far, so uncontroversial (I hope).

Next I turn to "an appreciation of science." I'll have more to say about this shortly, but for now let me simply report that I most definitely don't mean what you probably think I mean, which is anything like the current "standard science curriculum," where students are assessed on their ability to solve projectile problems or detail the likelihood of various chemical processes or define the function of ribosomes. In fact, while all of those things eventually need to be addressed for those keen to put themselves on the path to developing a more specialized understanding, the way science is typically taught—bombarding people with arbitrary and mind-numbingly boring arcana at the outset in a highly authoritarian way—is perhaps our single most flagrant educational failure: creating widespread public confusion about what science is and does while simultaneously repelling huge numbers of curious, talented would-be scientists from the field altogether. In short, if you were determined to create a society rife with deep misunderstanding of what science is all about, you'd be hard pressed to come up with a better instrument for doing so than most high school science curricula.

The whole thing is profoundly, mesmerizingly backwards. And Lewis Thomas, as usual, keenly diagnosed the situation decades earlier:

> *"I suggest that the introductory courses in science, at all levels from grade school through college, be radically revised. Leave the fundamentals, the so-called basics, aside for a while, and concentrate the attention of all students on the things that are not known...Do not teach that biology is a useful and perhaps profitable science; that can come later. Teach instead that there are structures squirming inside all our cells, providing all the energy for living, that are essentially foreign creatures, brought in for symbiotic living a billion or so years ago, the lineal descendants of bacteria.*

> *Teach that we do not have the ghost of an idea how they got there, where they came from, or how they evolved to their present structure and function. The details of oxidative phosphorylation and photosynthesis can come later."*[5]

Given that it is difficult to imagine a significant area of contemporary public policy that is completely independent of science, it is hardly an Einsteinian-level insight to conclude that if the overall goal is to generate a more productively-engaged citizenry, it's vital to ensure that they have a basic general understanding of what science is and how it works.

My third suggested area, "history of their country" is hardly without controversy, given the perennial, and often quite distorting, role that nationalistic propaganda has long played in public policy. But that's all the more reason, it seems to me, to insist that all citizens have a basic understanding and appreciation of not only what has occurred to shape their society, but also—far less stressed but equally if not more important—why.

An example might help to illustrate my thoughts here. Last year I published a little book[6] in which, along with other considerably more speculative assertions, I examined various popular misconceptions of contemporary American life, at one point launching myself into a detailed investigation of some of the more manifestly anti-democratic aspects of the US Constitution in order to illustrate the obvious falseness of the oft-touted claim that the United States of America was explicitly created as a democracy.

Now, most Americans are well aware of the existence of specific undemocratic attributes of their political framework—of which the

---

[5] "Humanities and Science" in *Late Night Thoughts on Listening to Mahler's Ninth Symphony*

[6] *Exceptionally Upsetting: How Americans are increasingly confusing knowledge with opinion & what can be done about it*

Electoral College is the most obvious example—but alarmingly few seem to have ever wondered *why* such things exists in the first place. And what I found particularly troubling is that it's actually not very hard to figure that out. The 1787 Constitutional Convention was an extremely clearly-defined historical event from which we have a comprehensive record of internal happenings,[7] together with a wealth of revealing correspondence of many of the leading protagonists. And a rapid perusal of this material quickly leads one to the indisputable conclusion that specific structural measures formulated in Philadelphia that summer, such as the Electoral College (as well as the original selection procedure of US Senators), were explicitly designed to be a *check* on democracy.

As always, one can take sides on whether this was a good thing or a bad thing, but the one conclusion that seems quite indefensible is to simply airbrush the whole thing away and blithely maintain the patently false claim that the architects of the US Constitution were uniformly determined to create the United States of America as a fully-fledged democracy. But that is, depressingly, precisely what has so often been done.

So yes, absolutely, let's insist upon a general awareness of national history. But by "history" I mean precisely that, not hand-waving mythologizing in striking contradistinction to the actual historical record.

The fourth category, a detailed understanding of how government works, is another area of study that is often already part of the general curriculum, with many countries having a type of "Civics" course where such topics are formally addressed. But just like "basic science" and "national history" the key question is, *Is it being done sufficiently well?* And it certainly doesn't look that way. In fact, several astute observers have remarked that, these days, it is increasingly not being done at all.

---

[7] The canonical text is Max Farrand's *The Records of the Federal Convention of 1787*, published in 1911 and freely available on many websites.

Paul Kahn for example, Robert W. Winner Professor of Law and the Humanities at Yale University, lamented that, far from meeting our fundamental societal needs, our current interest in Civics is clearly waning.

> *"Schools have given up teaching Civics as a necessary condition for a successful democracy. It's horrible that many schools treat it like religion today and just stay away from it."*

That alone, I think—the notion that schools are increasingly prone to regarding the teaching of the basic operations of government and the consequent rights and responsibilities of citizens as something akin to religious dogma—is nothing less than a bone-rattling alarm that your democratic project is in dire straits indeed.

It also brings to attention the sobering point that we all unhesitatingly accept that public education and daily politics will often collide, resulting in the frequent "politicization" of specific features of the school curriculum, such as the extent to which teaching evolution should be given equal billing with creationism.

Well, you might say, that's all part and parcel of living in a democracy: all public policy is subject to the machinations of politicians out to "leverage" matters for their own perceived political interest.

But this is not so. The reason that most countries have developed strict measures to ensure that their central banks can act independently from the government of the day is precisely because we have learned through painful experience that, left up to their own devices, politicians will invariably try to use the tools of monetary policy for their own short-term political ends, which are often distinctly contrary to those of the nation at large.

The successful implementation of prudent monetary policy, in other words, is universally recognized as being far too important to the nation's long-term interest to be needlessly subjected to inevitable political interests, so specific structural mechanisms have been created and implemented to protect its integrity. Education, meanwhile, one can't but conclude, is simply not viewed as important enough.

The final requirement on my list, an ability to assess claims and evaluate evidence, is, I'm convinced, the most important of the lot, implicitly referencing a point that I brought up several pages ago on the distinction between being educated and possessing knowledge. We've seen how the common perception that education is simply the process of pouring knowledge into students' heads and then testing them on their ability to recapitulate it is woefully misguided, giving them, among many other things, a deeply distorted view of science and a critically unreflective and often just plain incorrect understanding of history.

But that's only the beginning of your troubles. Because if you divide the world into distinct, non-overlapping camps of those who possess knowledge and those who don't, then there's no logically conceivable way that the vast majority of people can play any meaningful role in the formation of public policy, since they naturally won't have any specialized knowledge about the topic in question.

In fact, it's not just that most of your citizenry will be excluded—which is bad enough—it's that *everyone* will quickly be excluded. The only people who'd be qualified to formulate laws on climate change, say, would be professional climate scientists; and they, in turn, would naturally be incapable of weighing in on matters of health care or transportation policy or international relations or anything else. That's not the way it works; and it's not the way it can *possibly* work.

Here's Rush Holt, a member of the United States Congress for 16 years, describing how it actually works:

> *"As a Member of Congress, myself and the other 434 Representatives and 100 Senators were frequently confronted with issues that contained science; and even*

> *though we didn't know the details, we were able to evaluate whether or not a due process had been followed by the scientists who were presenting the technical information."*

As it happens, Rush was one of the few Congressmen over the past few decades who actually does have a scientific background, holding a PhD in physics. But the key point to emphasize is that he is not saying, *"Trust me: I'm qualified to make this decision because I have a PhD"*—but rather, *"It's the business of elected representatives to harness their general education skills in order to be able to confidently make decisions in areas where they do not personally hold specialized knowledge."*

Even more significantly, Rush vigorously maintains that precisely these same skills must be actively harnessed by the citizenry at large if the overall democratic project is to succeed.

> *"For democracy to work, for us to get to workable solutions, the public must be involved. And this also applies to scientific and technical issues that lie behind the decisions that governments make. It's quite possible—in fact, it frequently happens—that scientists are held accountable by non-scientists who ask, 'What's the evidence? Show us that you have arrived at these decisions in a way that removes bias from your conclusions, that your work has been openly critiqued and validated.'*
>
> *"Ordinary citizens can do this—I've seen it happen. It doesn't mean that every citizen has to do this on every decision. But on every decision there must be enough citizens, and enough citizen organizations, raising the questions and checking the process to hold the scientists accountable and get information that they are willing to trust and to use in the decision-making."*

How, precisely, can such generalized evaluative skills be taught? Is it reasonable to expect that a public education system can address this? I believe so, although it must be admitted in all candor that—ironically enough—there's a palpable dearth of evidence to support the claim.

The only high-school level program that I'm aware of that attempts to formally address this issue within a formalized educational framework is the so-called "Theory of Knowledge" course in the International Baccalaureate Diploma Program. I'd love to be able to report that it is a widespread success story and a worthy template for the sort of educational transformation that I'm calling for. But as far as I can tell that is hardly the case: the vast majority of teachers have no real understanding of its value and students correspondingly view it as little more than a minor, idiosyncratic diversion from their "real" academic trajectory. Still it exists, and thus serves as a concrete example to which we can point when discussing this issue.

Because for me, this is by far the most pressing educational concern that has been starkly brought to light by the pandemic: an alarmingly large number of people are incapable of making reasonable decisions. It is not so much that they are temporarily misinformed, believing X when Y is actually the case, or that they lack the necessary high-level expertise to navigate their way through the relevant details of a technical argument. And it is not that they are stupid. It is simply that they do not have the required skills to be able to sufficiently exercise their judgment. And these skills can be taught. But we are not doing so.

Once again: Since our societies have been deliberately structured so that the key decisions are dependent on the judgment of the citizenry at large, you'd think that the attempt to better cultivate their powers of judgment would be a top priority, and you certainly wouldn't think that any attempt to formally address this issue would be broadly considered to be "naive" or "Utopian" or "elitist." But you'd be wrong on both counts. And here we are.

Thus ends, rather depressingly, my K–12 thought experiment; and I found myself turning with considerable enthusiasm to the question of how our experience of the pandemic might somehow lead to improvements at the post-secondary level. This is, I recognize, a pretty strange statement in itself. The question of what the proper societal role of universities should be has been vigorously debated almost as long as its more generalized "basic educational" sibling, and has, on the whole, been just as ineffectual. So why the enthusiasm? Is it simply a case of anything being better than the prospect of trying to reformulate a public education curriculum?

Well, partly. But there are three other factors in play here.

The first is that universities, for all of their frequent incoherence, if not downright dysfunctionality, are largely self-contained, autonomous institutions—particularly if they have the good fortune to be private and well-endowed, as many of America's top institutions are—and thus the prospect that they might conceivably modify their behavior as a result of current circumstances is vastly less implausible than is the case for most high schools, let alone an entire "public educational system," notwithstanding any desperate analogies one might be tempted to put forth concerning the structural autonomy of central banks and so forth.

The second is that universities, being filled with older, more mature students who are there of their own free will, is notoriously a highly fertile ground for transformative social change.

But by far the biggest reason why I was particularly excited to be turning my attention to the pandemic's influence on universities was that it gave me a concrete opportunity to chat with Chris Celenza.

Chris is one of the world's experts on Renaissance humanism and has written widely, and extremely engagingly, on a number of topics from Petrarch to Machiavelli, provocatively combining questions of philology, philosophy, literary style, religion, politics and more to offer a riveting cultural anthropological depiction of what he calls "the long 15th century" of Renaissance Italy.

*Well*, I can imagine you saying, *that's all very nice, Howard, but what on earth does any of that have to do with the pandemic?* Truthfully, nothing. I suppose I could argue that I was intent on speaking with a scholar who was familiar with historical accounts of the devastation of the Black Death that ravaged Florence in 1348 in order to draw some penetrating parallels between how societies respond to plagues throughout the ages, but in fact I had no such intention and we never talked about that.[8]

But it came to my attention that, aside from constantly cranking out intriguing books on the Italian Renaissance, Chris also—quite inexplicably— regularly involves himself in academic administration; indeed, he is currently serving as Dean of Arts and Sciences at Johns Hopkins University.

Moreover, in his latest book, *The Italian Renaissance and the Origins of the Modern Humanities*, he makes a regular effort to connect the past with the present, often pausing to explicitly compare the "rapidly changing media landscape" of 15th-century Italy transformed by the new technology of movable type with our own, information-saturated age.

Given that the pandemic has dramatically increased our attention to how information and misinformation is being transmitted throughout society; and that, as the Dean of Arts and Sciences at one of the world's elite universities he would naturally be well-placed to discuss the impact of the pandemic on post-secondary institutions, it seemed that I had more than enough justification to contact him for this project.

And if, when all was said and done, he just wanted to hold forth on the merits of Marsilio Ficino, that would be fine with me too.

---

[8] As it happens, though, Teo Ruiz did—see chapter 8

But of course he had many penetrating and highly relevant things to say. He described how a decades-long diminution of trust in public institutions has been significantly exacerbated by the pandemic, declaring that:

> *"We need to do the best we can not to give the impression that we're just pronouncing on what's knowledge, we have to show people how we got there. We've got to get better at talking to the public not only about the work that we do but why we do it and how we do it."*

He admitted that students caught in the teeth of the pandemic had undergone a particularly difficult time, but speculated that on the whole they would likely emerge more resilient for the experience.

For me, however, his most thought-provoking comments concerned how the pandemic had given a major impetus to the necessity of changing both the student experience and the knowledge process itself.

> *"We must get away from the idea that students are passive recipients of knowledge that's generated elsewhere. Students have to become part of the enterprise of generating knowledge: they have to become knowledge-makers as well as knowledge-receivers."*

Lewis Thomas, I thought to myself, couldn't have said it better.

# 3. Appreciating Science

*"An appreciation of what is happening in science today, and of how great a distance lies ahead for exploring, ought to be one of the rewards of a liberal-arts education. Part of the intellectual equipment of an educated person, however his or her time is to be spent, ought to be a feel for the queerness of nature, the inexplicable things."*[1]

Talk to any scientist about the public perception of science and sooner or later the dreaded "answer at the back of the book" idiom will surface: the somehow unquenchable belief that everything substantial about nature is already known, or about to be known imminently. As Lewis Thomas describes it:

> *"The numbers are sitting out there in nature, waiting to be found, sorted and totted up. If only they had enough robots and enough computers, the scientists could go off to the beach and wait for their papers to be written for them; what we know about nature today is pretty much the whole story: we are very nearly home and dry. From here on, it is largely a problem of tying up loose ends, tidying nature up, getting the files in order."*[2]

This picture is, of course, patently absurd. Anyone who has the slightest familiarity with the actual scientific world is intimately aware of just

---

[1] "Humanities and Science" in *Late Night Thoughts on Listening to Mahler's Ninth Symphony*

[2] "Humanities and Science" in *Late Night Thoughts on Listening to Mahler's Ninth Symphony*

how much the frontiers of science, like the frontiers of anything, are replete with seemingly impenetrable mysteries, constantly-shifting conclusions, fierce debates, and a profound, almost paralyzing uncertainty about how to coherently proceed. And science, it should be stressed, has a whole lot of frontiers.

So why do so many so often get it so overwhelmingly wrong? Why does the "back of the book" perception of science continue to persist in the minds of so many people?

I'm not sure; but I have a few theories.

The first springs from comments in the previous chapter about the way science is typically taught. If your only detailed encounter with science consisted of being forced to address an array of standard problems, the answers to which could be found in the back of some book, it would hardly be unreasonable for you to conclude that performing such an activity is deeply reflective of what "science" actually is.

The exact same thing happens, and for precisely the same reason, when you try to convince people who have never taken a math course beyond the early undergraduate level (i.e. almost everyone) that, in striking contrast to all of their personal experience, the practice of mathematics is actually a deeply creative, highly intuitive activity practiced by those who are inexorably driven by a profound sense of aesthetics. They look at you as if you are completely off your rocker.

The second point is that, notwithstanding all the uncertainties and mysteries that amply surround us, science has worked extraordinarily well over the past few centuries. And so, while we should always be on our guard against the hubris of believing that we know much more than we actually do, engaging in the false modesty that we really don't know much at all when we've obviously learned an awful lot about a great many things clearly won't do either. There is considerable evidence, as it were, to have a great deal of confidence in the scientific process, broadly defined. While we're obviously a far cry from being able to find all the answers, that doesn't mean that we can't be quite confident of several insights that we've justifiably come to rely upon.

The third point is that it's necessary to say, "the scientific process, broadly defined," not just because specific research avenues use a panoply of different approaches, but because it is rarely far from obvious to know where exactly the boundary is between what is science and what is not, nor to what extent that is even a useful distinction at all.

While most of us are reasonably confident that a cosmologist is somehow, more or less, doing the same sort of thing as a geneticist, things get increasingly fuzzy as we move towards incorporating epidemiologists, say, in our categorization scheme; and by the time we reach economists, many of us—myself very much included—begin to suspect that it's high time we started over entirely. And it has long struck me as noteworthy that the further away people are from what might be immediately accepted as being "scientific," the more determined they seem to be to convince people that that's precisely where they belong. Which is all to say that, while perhaps not strictly promulgating a "back of the book" sort of dogma, there are definitely more than a few segments of the professional world that are swift to adopt the *"I'm a scientist (more or less), you can trust me"* tag line.

Which brings me, with a thud, to the hugely enraging exclamation that has been uttered with such astonishing frequency over the last two years: "Trust the Science!"

There is so much wrong with this sneeringly declarative statement that it is very difficult to know where exactly to begin attacking it, from the Enlightenment-distorting intimation that science is effectively equivalent to a form of religious faith; to the patently false assumption, that the line between "science" and "non-science" is always self-evidently razor-sharp, consistently cutting the world into two non-overlapping regions that are transparently obvious to anyone with a modicum of common sense, to the sulfurous whiff of the ad hominem demonization of one's adversaries as hidebound troglodytes whose lack of intellectual acuity should properly be pitied.

But worst of all, I think, is the dangerous implication that, as democratic citizens, our job is to summarily throw our trust in one direction or the other, as opposed to diligently invoking our critical power of judgment that I spent so much of the last chapter going on about in lurid detail.

Which is all to say that if I were somehow forced to choose between attending a "Trust the Science!" rally and a "Don't Trust the Science!" rally, I suppose I would begrudgingly plunk for the former, but I can assure you that it would be a close-run thing.

When confronted with this sort of reaction, most people will respond with something like, "*When we say, 'Trust the Science!' we really mean this business of using our critical faculties that you keep going on about. What we're saying is simply that it's important to use evidence-based approaches in our decision procedure as opposed to indulging in mere wishful thinking and/or simply giving free reign to our biases.*"

Now, I get that, of course—indeed, it is the principal reason why, if push came to shove, I'd opt to attend the "Trust the Science!" rally over the "Don't Trust the Science!" rally—but if that is what you are really trying to say, then you should just say that, even if it means having to work much harder to find a way to make your message fit into a pithy slogan on the signs you are determined to be waving around (or simply be prepared to bring along bigger signs). Otherwise you risk doing far more harm than good to the cause of "communicating science" that you are trying so hard to convince me you are so fiercely dedicated to.

Because the truth is that the issues raised by this sort of inquiry—What *is* science, exactly? Where do we draw the line?—are complex, subtle, historically significant, and very much worth paying attention to.

Take it from Princeton University historian of science Michael Gordin, who has devoted considerable time and effort to plumbing the intriguing divide between "science" and "pseudoscience," writing two books on the topic[3] filled with an array of insights that are often just as valuable for "established scientists" as those who find themselves on the "fringe" enviously looking in.

In particular, it's very common to hear a practicing scientist unhesitatingly declare that the distinction between science and pseudoscience is an obvious one, long-sorted out by Karl Popper in the early 20th century. The corresponding historical context, Michael explains, is as follows:

> *"At the time, the dominant philosophical school in Vienna was Logical Positivism, which had a very strong tradition of verificationism: that is, science is science because it finds things that verify itself against nature. Popper thinks that's not true, because he believes that one can always find verifying instances, or at least interpret them as verifying instances. What he wants instead is what he came to call 'falsificationism.' He says, Something is scientific when it says, 'If you find this, I'm wrong,' In other words, it's not about being right. It's about not being wrong **yet**."*[4]

It seems very straightforward. And years ago when I was running a research institute it was very common to encounter physicists unhesitatingly invoking the merits of "falsifiability" all the time—indeed, I expect it happens just as frequently today. But on careful reflection, it turns out to be considerably more problematic than first meets the eye, with three significant issues associated with it.

> *"Problem one is, How do you know that you've falsified something? If it were the case that every time an experiment*

---

[3] *The Pseudoscience Wars: Immanuel Velikovsky and the Birth of the Modern Fringe* and *On the Fringe: Where Science Meets Pseudoscience*

[4] This quote and the one following is taken from chapter 8 of *Science and Pseudoscience–A Conversation with Michael Gordin*

*with a null result meant that you'd falsified something, then everything we know about physics and chemistry would be wrong because high school students around the world have failed to replicate it. So you have to do the experiment right. But how do you know you've done the experiment 'right' unless you get 'the right result'?*

"*Problem two is that any valuable demarcation criterion has to cut the world in the right place. That is, we want to make sure that all the things that we regard as science are scientific, and those things that we think of as 'fringe' or 'pseudo' are not. But the problem is that there are lots of types of science which have a very hard time coming up with falsifying instances: in particular, the historically-engaged sciences like evolutionary theory, geology, cosmology and so forth. You can't rerun the tape. If someone tells you, 'The universe was created this way,' it's awfully hard to find a falsifiable statement associated with that.*

"*The third problem with Popper's criterion is more of a philosophical one: it requires you to not believe in truth. Consistently applying it means that nothing is ever true: scientists make no true claims. I can't say, 'This chair is made of atoms.' I can only say, 'No one has disproved the claim that this chair is made of atoms **yet**.' It's a very uncomfortable position to be in in the long term.*"

The fact that we can't always unthinkingly invoke some reliable algorithm to distinguish between science and pseudoscience doesn't mean, of course, that all claims are equivalent or that there's no way to ever make meaningful judgments about anything, or that we have to definitively abandon the word "science" from our vocabularies. It simply means that on the whole things are a good deal more complex and nuanced than many people would have us believe—a sort of general truism that applies to a wide range of phenomena, as general truisms are wont to do—and is thus all the more reason for us to carefully develop our critical faculties so as to be able to repeatedly apply them on a case by case basis. So we're back to that once again, I fear.

It also means that battles over "trust," "authority" and "evidence" will always be with us, and we should not be surprised when lines are crossed on all sides, as they often are, particularly in the white heat of a raging pandemic when there's a natural conviction that *something* must be done, and quickly.

But there are, I think, two other important implications of the structural inability to distinguish between "science" and "non-science," that bear commenting on.

The first is that "appreciating science" throughout broader society should really not be as difficult as it is often made out to be. After all, if it actually were the case that science was a fundamentally different sort of activity that was engaged in by fundamentally different types of people—robot-like calculators, presumably, who waltzed through life confidently expecting that the answers to all of their questions could be found in the back of some book somewhere—then it would naturally be very challenging for the rest of us to develop any sort of comprehension of the scientific enterprise or empathy for those who do it, given how our own lives are so contrastingly filled with uncertainty, ambiguity, missteps, serendipitous insights, false hopes, profound surprises and wonder.

But once we are reassured that science is a human endeavor just like poetry or metalworking or storytelling, we will naturally expect such things to be part and parcel of the scientific enterprise too. Moreover, we will also not be amazed to discover that features often exclusively associated with "the scientific method"—the construction and testing of hypotheses, the painstaking search for past precedents and confirming instances, the development of theoretical frameworks—are frequently incorporated into a great many outlooks and attitudes that are not customarily or primarily regarded as "scientific." I've often ruefully wondered how many judges or historians or literary theorists have found themselves utterly bemused by the common equivalence between "evidence-based" and "scientific" that is bandied about everywhere these days. What, in god's name, do people think these guys are doing all day long?

So that's one point that you wouldn't think needed to be made, but somehow seems to be: since science is a human activity, its human practitioners do it in order to fulfill basic human desires. That this comes as a shock to many other humans is yet another mystery that one can only hope scientific inquiry might one day shed light on.

But slightly less obviously, it works the other way around too. For once it is recognized that there is no impenetrable divide between "scientific" and "non-scientific" matters, there is a drastically increased possibility that what was hitherto not officially recognized as "scientific" might actually be of use to scientists.

And by that I don't mean the sorts of things that are usually invoked when people talk about how most scientists would benefit from exposure to external activities, like music or football or gardening, so as to be able to interact better with their neighbors or live more balanced lives.

That's doubtless true too, but what I'm talking about here is how exposing members of the scientific community to a range of broader influences and perspectives can directly aid the understanding of *science itself*, which is a strikingly different sort of claim, and one that is heard much less frequently. But it likely won't surprise you by now to learn that Lewis Thomas has said as much on several occasions.

In "How to Fix the Premedical Curriculum,"[5] this former Dean of Yale Medical School recommended, only slightly tongue in cheek, that the very category of "premedical student" should be officially eliminated,

---

[5] In *The Medusa and the Snail*

that classical Greek should be restored as the centerpiece of undergraduate education, and that, *"English, history, the literature of at least two foreign languages, and philosophy should come near the top of the list, just below Classics as basic requirements; and applicants for medical school should be told that their grades in these courses will count more than anything else."*

Why? The students themselves, he averred, would be the primary beneficiaries, given that they would no longer be singled out as belonging to the premeds—*"that most detestable of all cliques eating away at the heart of the college,"* followed by the college faculties who would find themselves, *"once again in possession of the destiny of their own curriculum, for better or worse."* All very amusing, you might think. But then this:

> *"Perhaps benefiting most of all are the basic-science faculties of the medical schools, who would once again be facing classrooms of students who are ready to be startled and excited by a totally new and unfamiliar body of knowledge, eager to learn, unpreoccupied by the notions of relevance that are paralyzing the minds of today's first-year medical students already so surfeited by science that they want to start practicing psychiatry in the first trimester of the first year."*

Well, you might say, medical students are not, by and large, really scientists anyway—a fair point to which we shall return in chapter 9—but Thomas goes on to give several other telling examples, such as his penetrating analysis of Lord Kelvin's erroneous calculation of the age of the earth and solar system, which produced a date much too late for evolution to have significantly occurred on the scale that it needed to, thereby provoking widespread consternation among biologists, Darwin most definitely included.[6]

---

[6] See "Humanities and Science" in *Late Night Thoughts on Listening to Mahler's Ninth Symphony*

Kelvin, an indisputably great scientist, had earlier opined, *"When you can measure what you are speaking about, and express it in numbers, you know something about it. But when you cannot—your knowledge is of a meager and unsatisfactory kind."*

But, Thomas warns us:

> *"As at least one subsequent event showed, Kelvin may have had things exactly the wrong way round. The task of converting observations into numbers is the hardest of all, the last task rather than the first thing to be done, and it can be done only when you have learned, beforehand, a great deal about the observations themselves."*

Anyone who has done any computer modeling has an intuitive understanding of what is being expressed here. It's often summed up by the phrase "garbage in, garbage out": no matter how fancy your mathematical simulation, if you are not actually modeling what is really going on in the world—if your understanding of the core processes at play is incomplete, or you are inserting unreliable data into your initial conditions (or, as often occurs, some combination of the two)—then whatever your model spits out at the end of the day isn't worth a damn.

And we've seen this time and again during the coronavirus pandemic. If you don't have a clear sense of how the virus is actually transmitted, or you don't properly take into account the high levels of asymptomaticity associated with COVID-19, or you don't actually have any good sense of the numbers of people who are currently infected in a given region or set of regions—let alone when all three errors are occurring at once—then your epidemiological model is not producing any "trustworthy science" whatsoever, no matter how powerful the computer you are running it with or how confidently you are asserting your results or how prestigious your academic post.

In Kelvin's case, he had made his calculations based upon an extrapolation of the fundamental physical processes as understood at the time—an understanding that was, unbeknownst to him, going to be comprehensively revolutionized in relatively short order. Of course, he couldn't possibly have foreseen this at the time, and the unprecedented waves of progress characterized by 19th-century physics gave him every reason to be confident. Which was, Thomas pointedly summarizes, ironically enough the very crux of the problem:

> *"The system for gaining information and comprehension about nature works so well, indeed, that it carries another hazard: the risk of convincing yourself that you know everything."*

Given all of this, it is particularly shocking that most practicing scientists have little to no regard for the value of the history of science. While some might read a few books on the subject out of interest, the vast majority have not been exposed to any level of formal historical training beyond high school (and sometimes not even there). As we can be quite confident that human beings have not evolved substantially since modern science began, this strikes me as a particularly toxic combination of hubris and obduracy: a deep-rooted, thoroughly unreflective, evidence-free conviction that centuries of potentially meaningful insights have nothing to teach us, that mastering any particular operational technique is vastly more relevant to solving any contemporary scientific challenge than making the effort to piece together an understanding of what other thoughtful people, in broadly similar situations, have done and with what results.

We are, to put it in scientific terms, needlessly ignoring centuries of highly valuable data. Talk about a lack of appreciation.

# 4. Making Decisions

> *"In real life, this is the way we've always arrived at decisions, even though it has always been done in a disorganized way. We pass the word around; we ponder how the case is put by different people; we read the poetry; we meditate over the literature; we play the music; we change our minds; we reach an understanding. Society evolves this way, not by shouting each other down, but by the unique capacity of unique, individual human beings to comprehend each other."*[1]

Whenever I mentioned how I was interested in using the COVID-19 crisis as a vehicle to examine our democratic decision-making processes, people would inevitably assume that I was intent on comparing the effectiveness of emergency health policies in democratic and nondemocratic countries, or that I was keen to use the pandemic to examine the pernicious effects of populism.

But that's not the sort of thing I had in mind. While I anticipated that particular aspects of those issues, along with many others, would inevitably arise, my principal goal—on a conceptual par with chapter 2's question, To what extent could it reasonably be maintained that we actually live in a "well-educated society"?—was much more general: *What does our response to the pandemic reveal about the strengths and weaknesses of our governance structures?*

The biggest problem with asking questions like, *Are democracies doing a better job fighting the pandemic than autocratic regimes?* or *How has the pandemic exacerbated populism?* is that, for the most part, they

---

[1] "On Committees" in *The Medusa and the Snail*

aren't really questions at all. You already have a clear idea in your head of what the answer should be: democracies are good, autocratic regimes are bad, and everyone knows which is which; and if it turns out that some of the numbers temporarily seem to favor obviously undemocratic regimes that is only because the numbers are false, or they don't tell the whole story, or they are only related to short-term effects, or the pandemic turns out to be the exception that proves the rule, or whatever. Similarly for populism, a term that is almost always invoked in a deliberately hand-waving way as an opaque synonym for a sadly unavoidable mechanism that places the wrong sort of people in power.

It is not that I am a champion of either autocracy or those generally regarded as populist politicians these days (it is safe to say that I am neither), but the whole point of the exercise is to move well and truly beyond tautological projections of current beliefs and instead, as always, concentrate on how we might use the pandemic as a lens to probe what the hell is really going on. And to do that, it seems to me, you naturally have to turn inwards: harnessing this pivotal moment to examine, as honestly and rigorously as you can, the strengths and weaknesses of your own governance structures (which are clearly the only ones that we can make any genuine claim to having any detailed understanding of).

The goal, in short, is simply to find a way to do better: to frankly acknowledge and understand our shortcomings so that we might discover how to ameliorate them in the future. If you are an American, the phrase "more perfect Union" might well spring to mind at this point. The rest of us, meanwhile, can simply content ourselves with "common sense."

Whenever I find myself particularly frustrated by the vapidly ahistorical, superficial cant about contemporary politics that the chattering classes are constantly spewing forth (which is often) and wish to produce some Ideas Roadshow content on the topic that might in some tiny way serve as a potential corrective (which is not), I turn to John Dunn.

John is an eminent political theorist at the University of Cambridge and widely regarded as one of the world's foremost authorities on John Locke. He has also written extensively on the history of democracy, carefully examining numerous applications, misapplications, strengths, weaknesses, successes, failures, truths, distortions and much more besides that have been done in its name. His writings are not always the easiest to grapple with—his style is replete with sinewy, unremittingly long sentences (yes, yes, I know: who am I to judge?)—but they are always very much worth the effort. He has much to say, does John. And I only wish that more people would listen.

As usual, when I approached him for this project, he quickly agreed. And as usual, he didn't disappoint:

> *"It isn't just that democracy isn't a guarantee of a secure and good collective life; it's that it can't be anything but a serious **menace** to the prospects for such a life except insofar as the citizens perform at a much higher level than they've so far learned how to."*

This is, I think, a most appropriate place to begin our investigations, forcing us to abruptly discard the standard cliché-riddled phrasebook, where obvious geopolitical self-interest is regularly passed off as deep moral sensitivity[2] and dig a bit deeper.

In other words, just telling ourselves that we live in a democracy so everything will necessarily be OK, does nothing. It is, as Wolfgang Pauli

---

[2] The photo of the recent American "Summit for Democracy" that was inserted into John's film clip was not, suffice it to say, a coincidence.

memorably expressed in another very different context, "not even wrong."[3]

Whether or not things will turn out well in the end naturally depends on the decisions we make. And if we want to do our best to ensure that, on the whole, we are making the best sorts of decisions, we have to convince ourselves that the specific decision-making processes we've put in place are functioning as well as possible.

In a democracy, those decision-making processes naturally depend, to some extent at least, on the broader citizenry—which is why John singles out an improved "performance" on their part as a necessary condition for progress, and a lack of improvement as little less than a recipe for disaster.

But what, actually, does this "performance" entail? To what extent might our current structural mechanisms be enhancing or inhibiting the prospects of its improvement—or, rather more subtly, the prospects of the citizenry somehow learning how to improve their performance? Perhaps, I wondered, our response to the pandemic might be able to shed some valuable light on that.

Of course, it might also be the case that it won't. It is perfectly conceivable, in fact, that a careful examination of how we are responding to an urgent, exceptional crisis is more of a distraction to addressing those sorts of general issues than any sort of "illuminating window." Or perhaps it will turn out to be a bit of both, with regular vigilance needed to successfully parse things out. Time will tell.

But before we take a detailed plunge into investigating the mechanics of public policy related to the pandemic—how decisions were reached, who was involved, and how effective or ineffective they were—it's worth pausing a moment to explicitly consider the question of who,

---

[3] I'm likely going to use this quote at least one more time in this book: it is an unavoidable thing to be doing whenever one engages in social commentary. Just ask Peter Woit.

exactly, are the objects of such public policy. For whom are we making these decisions anyway?

I appreciate that this question might well strike you as so obvious as to be borderline nonsensical. Surely objects of public policy are simply the public, no? The targets of Italian public policy are Italian citizens, the targets of Swedish public policy are Swedish citizens, and so forth. There doesn't seem to be much in the way of a profound mystery there.

But there is, I think, an important subtlety at play, the glimmers of which first dawned on me as I listened to Paul Kahn discussing his sense of democracy's basic requirements.

"*Democracy thrives in a community of care*," he announced, before pointing out in some detail how the most troubling characteristic of contemporary American life is that its two main political communities don't seem to genuinely care about each other at all.

When I first heard this I thought that the key point had to do with "societal values," unthinkingly slotting his comments into my envisioned chapter on what the crisis revealed about our shifting sense of collective morality.[4] The American response to the pandemic, went the argument, vividly highlighted the steadily mounting prepandemic concern that Americans had somehow lost their collective powers of empathy. Why was that? What was going on?

On reflection, I couldn't help sensing that my focus on a lack of empathy wasn't exactly wrong, but was somehow incomplete, glossing over a vital link in the conceptual chain. I had a nagging feeling that something important was being overlooked, but I couldn't quite figure out what.

Thankfully, Paul kept going:

---

[4] See chapter 8

> *"John Dewey, asked why we don't have a civil war after every election. After all, the majority wins and the minority is defeated. What is it that binds the minority to the electoral outcome?"*

A similar question, he noted, applies to a judicial decision, where everyone agrees to accept the final verdict in advance. Why? Because it is intuitively understood that every member of both the majority and the minority belong to the same community and are thus structurally in a position of caring for each other.

Suddenly, I thought of a memorable discussion I had years ago with the renowned intellectual historian Quentin Skinner where he was describing his efforts to puzzle out a historically significant understanding of "freedom" that was quite different from what we mean by that term today. According to this view, Quentin explained, being "free" meant something quite different than our contemporary notion of simply being left alone to do what we wanted, but was instead a form of *status*: a recognition that you were a member of a community where the governing laws were not arbitrarily imposed on you from without, but rather faithfully reflected the collective will of the community of which you were a participating member. By this measure, a "free person" was then someone who actively participated in the development of those laws, while those who had no role in their creation but were simply subjected to having these laws externally imposed upon them, were correspondingly regarded as "slaves."

Well, I began thinking to myself, perhaps the question isn't so much a lack of empathy per se, as a suddenly shifted perception of what one's proper "community" really is. After all, if I live in Greece, I don't really care what sorts of laws people in Norway are passing. And that hardly implies that I lack empathy or that I hate Norwegians. It's just that what's happening in Norway is straightforwardly and quite reasonably recognized as not being directly relevant to me. It's not my community. So if the government of Greece would suddenly inform me that for the next few months my actions would be subjected to Norwegian laws,

I'd be justifiably indignant, regardless of whether I believed those laws were appropriate or not. In fact, chances are that I wouldn't even bother considering the intrinsic merits or demerits of those laws at all; my immediate reaction would be something like, *Why on earth should I subject myself to laws that aren't ours?*

And similarly, if I live in West Virginia, say, and get word that those in New York or California have opted to invoke a series of strict measures against the pandemic that I strongly disagree with, my reaction might be to shrug my shoulders. But if you then told me that, for some reason over which I had no apparent control, my community would be subjected to those very same measures, it's not terribly surprising that all hell would break loose.

Now, I appreciate that the instinctive response to this is to cry out that the structural relationship of West Virginia to California—or, perhaps more relevantly, West Virginia to Washington D.C.—is significantly different from that of Greece to Norway, given that West Virginia, California and Washington D.C. are part of the same country and Greece and Norway are not. But then, perhaps things have now reached a point where the parallel is, in fact, much stronger than we have hitherto appreciated, with the pandemic helping to reveal that the standard claim, "But they're both part of the same (national) community!" is actually much less obviously meaningful than we might have instinctively supposed. There is, after all, no one clearly defined Platonic Form for what is, or is not, a "community." Once members of a collective no longer view themselves as being part of it, then they aren't. And once significant numbers of members feel that way the scope and scale of that collective is inevitably altered.

When faced with a rapidly changing community, when confronted with a situation where large numbers of people who used to self-identify with one group no longer feel motivated to do so, the obvious thing to wonder is what might have happened to prompt such a change. Did the core values of large numbers of members suddenly shift? If so, why, exactly? And how? Or perhaps it is a mirage. Perhaps the result isn't so much the fact that core personal values have spontaneously altered as the fact that many have become falsely convinced that something like that has occurred, the inevitable result of a vigorous misinformation campaign to persuade people that they no longer rightfully belonged to a community that they once felt inextricably attached to? If so, why? And by whom?

Good questions all—some of which, perhaps, we might develop some deeper understanding of as these investigations progress. But for now let's return to the matter at hand, which is to examine to what extent—if at all—our recent experiences of grappling with this uniquely intense public health crisis might serve as a valuable prism to critically examine to what extent our public policy mechanisms are both well-constructed and effective.

A most useful starting point, I think, is provided by Michael Frazer, Associate Professor of Political and Social Theory at the University of East Anglia. In the fall of 2016 I had an enjoyable filmed conversation[5] with Michael on his work on the so-called "Sentimentalist Enlightenment" of David Hume, Adam Smith and others. That convinced me that he's naturally predisposed to stepping back and taking a synoptic, "big picture" view of things that such an overarching analysis naturally requires. And so he promptly did.

> *"The issue of legitimacy has always been central to politics—the question of who has the right to rule and why—with two of the best candidates for legitimacy being rule by the people and rule by the experts.*
>
> *"The classic way to reconcile these competing claims, both of which seem valid, is through widespread public enlightenment. And the people don't need that high a level of expertise to*

---

[5] *The Power of Sympathy: Politics and Moral Sentimentalism–A Conversation with Michael Frazer*

> *make the right decisions. Condorcet's jury theorem proves they each just need slightly more than 50% chance of being correct for a majority vote to result in the right decision.*
>
> *"But the experience of the pandemic has led many to doubt this traditional solution to the problem, because in communities where misinformation is widespread, this average individual threshold will not be reached and a majority vote will guarantee an incorrect decision."*

This clearly poses a real and pressing concern to our decision-making practices. But the solution, Michael assures us, is most definitely not to simply ridicule people for their lack of expertise, which is inherently counterproductive:

> *"Even if the ignorant ought to cede to the rule of experts, at least on the subjects on which they're ignorant, if the experts and their allies just mock and dismiss them they will not do so."*

A few weeks later Rush Holt emphatically reinforced this sentiment by insisting that:

> *"No amount of scientific expertise is a substitute for public engagement, since the goal is not to get 'the right answer,' but to get 'workable answers.' And 'workable answers' depend on the involvement of the governed."*

This is a point that the pandemic demonstrates with stunning forcefulness. It doesn't matter how high the efficacy rates of your vaccine are, or how quickly you bring it to market, or how comprehensively you can manage to distribute it amongst the population. If significant numbers of people won't take it, then you don't have an effective solution to the problem.

Politics is not a theoretical exercise, it is a practical activity. The very notion of "the best possible solution" that is envisioned at the outset necessarily incorporates the assumption that such a solution can actually be implemented. It is not enough to know what to do (which is often hard enough), it is essential that whatever is eventually decided upon is broadly endorsed throughout society.

There are various different perspectives on how this could happen. Some insist that the key lies with developing high levels of trust in elected representatives. If the people can be somehow assured that their representatives are acting with their best interests in mind, goes the argument, they will naturally accept their recommendations.

Others, like Rush, believe the key is to somehow incorporate citizen organizations in the development of decisions right from the beginning, thereby ensuring that the citizenry has a tangible way to "buy in" throughout the entire process.

Then there are those who are convinced that the most necessary feature to emphasize is transparency: shining a light on the internal workings of policymaking so that the public can watch the decision-making process in action and learn what specific chain of reasoning led to the adoption of any particular measure.

But University of Exeter philosopher John Dupré looks at things slightly differently, focusing his attention on how our modern interpretation of "representation" bears considerable responsibility for much of our current state of political malaise.

> *"We are currently living in a very extreme form of populist democracy, by which I mean a democracy in which politicians represent the people not in the classical sense that thinkers like J.S. Mill believed they should—by being the people you want to think for you and make decisions—but by being the people who exactly think what you think."*

Three things stand out from John's comments. The first is that, by going to the trouble of actually defining what he means by "populist," he provides us with a revealing avenue to specifically analyze the structural issues at play, as opposed to indulging in the usual formulaic, dismissive invocation of populism to indicate personal political dissatisfaction.

The second is the recognition that the solution to our current problems cannot simply be "more democracy," because whatever its faults might be, the framework of picking representatives on the basis that "they think exactly what you think" cannot coherently be assailed as being "anti-democratic." Indeed, there is a clear case to be made that such an outlook is, logically, inherently *more* democratic than, say, John Stuart Mill's notion that representatives should be selected primarily based upon their character, experience and general probity.

Lastly, there is a clear link implied between who is involved in the decision-making process and what they are expected to be doing in that process.

If it is universally understood that participants have been selected simply on the basis of how faithfully they mirror the perceived will of their constituents, the most significant concern for them will naturally be to ensure that any action they take will be unhesitatingly endorsed by those constituents, which will inevitably lead to them acting in accordance with whatever the poll of the moment indicates, together with the near-constant occurrence of such polls.

If, on the other hand, it is generally recognized that those involved in forming policy are there because they have particularly well-developed decision-making skills, then they will naturally feel compelled to give priority to the exhibition of such skills in the usual sorts of ways—weighing evidence, exposing themselves to the widest variety of relevant perspectives, listening to contrary opinions and so forth.

And one particular benefit of using the coronavirus pandemic as the instance to probe the functioning of our decision-making systems is that it is hard to envision a situation where the utilization of broad-based investigatory skills is more paramount. When arguing over the policy details of an issue that has been carefully studied for decades, it is doubtless advisable to try to go the extra mile to see if you can uncover something new, but it is a pretty safe bet to assume that most people won't actually do so.

But when you're facing a crisis the likes of which you've never seen before, forced to choose between a number of hugely unpalatable emergency measures based upon a welter of recommendations from an array of experts with little to no understanding of anything outside of their own highly specialized domain (and, moreover, who are clearly relying on incomplete data and a fuzzy mechanistic understanding even there), it's a rather different kettle of fish altogether.

There are times, in other words, when you can muddle through in politics, never feeling truly obliged to roll up your intellectual sleeves and find solutions to best safeguard the health and welfare of those who chose you to look out for their interests. The COVID-19 pandemic isn't one of them.

Which brings me to Alexandre Quintanilha, an active Member of the Portuguese Parliament who had, and continues to have, a first-hand look at how the government of Portugal handled its response to the pandemic. He is also, as it happens, an internationally-acclaimed biologist[6] and a deeply thoughtful and reflective fellow. In short, it is hard to imagine someone better placed to meaningfully comment on what our experiences grappling with the pandemic might have taught us, politically speaking.

---

[6] Alex was the longtime director of the Institute of Molecular and Cell Biology at the University of Porto

Alex was naturally anxious to share specific lessons learned from the Portuguese government's response to the pandemic, but before he did so he took a moment to highlight a vital feature of this particular crisis that most people hadn't fully appreciated but one that he was particularly qualified to comment on: the significant cultural gap between the scientific and political domains and the consequent difficulty of bridging the two in real time during an emergency.

> *"It's a difficult balancing act: the generation of knowledge takes time, yet politics requires action and doesn't have the luxury of time. So trying to balance the careful accumulation of new scientific knowledge with how governments act is not easy."*

Many people, he explained, make a false equivalence between "data,, "information" and "knowledge"; somehow assuming that they are all different expressions for the same thing. But they aren't.

> *"Knowledge isn't just data. Data has to be selected in order to become information; information has to be digested in order to become knowledge. And if we're lucky—and it doesn't happen all the time—we gain some wisdom out of the entire experience."*

There is much worth pondering here that has a direct bearing on our general thoughts about the decision-making process, not least of which being the notion of "selection." Once again, it is not enough to be mindlessly chanting "Listen to the science!" or even "Listen to the data!" because the obvious response is: *Which science? What data?* Formulating appropriate policy requires a constant vigilance that you are not only thoughtfully and critically "listening to the experts," but that you are constantly reflecting upon which experts need to be paid attention to in the first place.

It's not just a case of establishing who are the "bonafide experts" and who are not—which is usually not terribly difficult to do—or even figuring out which ones are offering the most trustworthy and prudent analysis of the current situation at any given moment—which is invariably much more difficult—it's also ensuring that you have not overlooked people or even entire disciplines very much worth paying attention to.

I'll return to this point shortly, but first let's hear from Alex on why he thinks that the Portuguese experience at dealing with the coronavirus pandemic has been "a success story," and what lessons he believes it holds for all of us.

> *"It has to do with trust. The government did something which I think ought to be reproduced everywhere: it convened weekly public meetings between members of the government and a wide variety of experts to look at the data and try to understand what we were getting from other parts of the world. And this was usually shown on TV, where those present would answer questions from the media.*
>
> *"I think this was a very, very important step. It made sure that the general public was aware that there was dialogue, but even more importantly that sometimes some questions didn't have answers. There were some issues that we simply didn't know the answer to and we had to be clear about that. We had to be clear about having to adopt certain strategies that might have to be reversed in the light of possible future data."*

Yet again there is much food for thought here, from the role of the media to the need for transparency in government deliberations. But for me the most salient point Alex makes is how the candid admission of ignorance by public representatives is a principal requirement for the development of public trust.

The assumption that pervades much of modern political life is precisely the opposite: that the worst thing any politician can say is "I don't know." Making such an admission, we are repeatedly told, is the veritable "third rail" of politics, immediately opening up an elected representative to vitriolic denouncements of incompetence and negligence that palpably demonstrate that she is "not fit to hold the public trust."

Far better instead, goes the thinking, to say something—anything—to desperately try to allay the suspicion that you might not actually be certain of what to do: confidently assure people that the crisis will pass, or sing the praises of a miraculous drug that you've vaguely heard of or portray your opponents as irredeemable worrywarts desperate to announce that the sky is falling. Or perhaps all three. It doesn't really matter what you say, in fact (after all, they likely won't remember the details anyway), all that counts is that you do it confidently and with sufficient authority to calm people down and give them the impression that you are a "strong leader" who will take care of them.

Except, of course, that doing so doesn't take care of them at all, which is hardly surprising given that your justification for saying such things was solely motivated by how you could best take care of *yourself*, through the careful protection of your own perceived public image.

I have never understood how this approach—how resolutely denying one's ignorance despite an abundance of evidence to the contrary—can be a successful political strategy. But it is undeniable that it is. Which is, I think, very important to appreciate. It is no use blaming media companies or communication strategists or corporate donors for the fact that politicians are inclined to adopt patently duplicitous strategies to retain public office. They do so because such strategies seem to work. The obvious question is, Why?

I wish I knew. But it is wonderful to contemplate that there are at least some places on earth where they don't. It's time for all of us, perhaps, to seriously consider moving to Portugal.

But before doing that there's one final point to touch on. Recall that a few moments ago, I referred to yet another decision-making complication that has been conspicuously illustrated by the pandemic.

Even if you have a well-established collective that consistently recognizes that the principal job of its governing institutions is to make decisions in the direct interests of the entire community; and even if you establish appropriate decision-making structures that palpably demonstrate that policy is being made in a transparent and duly deliberative manner, harnessing the highest level of domain-specific expertise that can be brought to bear on the issues at hand, there are still occasions when you will have to grapple with yet another concern: which *sorts* of expert domains should you consider including at the outset?

Not all issues necessarily have this additional component to them. If your attention is exclusively focused on quickly developing a vaccine, say, then you simply concentrate on finding and working with top professionals in the public and private sectors who are best placed to make that happen.

But what if, in the meantime, you are considering implementing an unprecedentedly large lockdown to limit the spread of the disease? Undoubtedly you will want to confer with virologists and epidemiologists who can proffer their expert opinions on which sorts of quarantine measures will be the most effective at reducing transmission of the pathogen, but equally certainly you should be doing your utmost to involve the widest spectrum of relevant domains to best assess the enormously broad impact any such policy will inevitably have. Well, that's the theory, anyway.

But as University of Indiana philosopher and cognitive scientist Ann-Sophie Barwich points out, all too often things don't actually work out that way; and they certainly didn't when it came to the decision to impose lockdowns.

> *"I think the most surprising aspect of the pandemic for me was to what extent there was this huge gap between our understanding of human cognition and the brain and the actual policies that were implemented.*
>
> *"We've seen, for instance, how social isolation elicits reactions in the human brain that resemble hunger and starvation. We also know that placing people together in the same room and involving them in the same task leads to an alignment of neural oscillations. The human brain is really a social organ.*
>
> *"But then we had this policymaking that suddenly put people into complete isolation without any real consideration of what that might mean for human cognition, interaction and the development of humans—especially young children who need social interaction in order to find themselves.*
>
> *"So, while you often hear things like, 'We're formulating evidence-based policy based on science,' it's clearly the case that there's been a lot of science that hasn't been included, and that gap needs to be bridged."*

And Ann-Sophie was hardly the only person to notice this sort of disconnect. Many of her sentiments were resoundingly echoed by renowned University of Queensland social psychologist Roy Baumeister as he described the disproportionately high toll that economically disruptive policies are known to take on society's younger people.

> *"We know from the Great Depression a century ago that the people most affected are those whose careers are at that critical point, typically in one's 30s. If there's a serious economic downturn, the effect of the downturn is temporary for society, but it's permanent for you if you miss out on the chance, because by the time the economy recovers there are new people coming along."*

Moreover, Roy told me, you can't always neatly separate health consequences into distinct, non-overlapping categories of "psychological" and "physical." Aside from the well-documented fact that one's mental state often has a clear causal impact on one's body (and vice-versa), there's a growing body of research that points to a dangerously significant impact of the lockdown on a community's death rate.

> *"There's even evidence that, when it comes to health matters, the effects of the lockdown are greater than the direct effects of the virus itself. Even in places that don't have a lot of COVID-related deaths, the death rate has gone up for a number of reasons, including reckless driving and abstention from preventative medical treatment. A lot of researchers have looked at this increased death rate closely and concluded that COVID had some effect on the numbers, but mostly on older, sick people; whereas the lockdown is affecting the entire population, including younger people."*

None of this is to definitely conclude, of course, that lockdowns were always counterproductive or should never have been imposed. That is far too pat a reaction, and once more harkens back to a dangerously unhelpful tendency to make all-encompassing, universal declarations that so demonstrably don't fit the complex, multivariable world in which we live.

Instead, the appropriate conclusion is simply to be ever-vigilant against the manifold dangers of hubris. When you're faced with an unfamiliar, highly dangerous, hugely unpredictable crisis that urgently calls for some sort of immediate action, it's essential to step back and deliberately involve the widest possible array of potentially relevant experts in the decision procedure, secure in the knowledge that doing so is the only reasonable approach to take given your current state of ignorance.

For Lewis Thomas, recognizing what we don't know was a necessary requirement to unlock future scientific breakthroughs. For those tasked with developing appropriate public policy measures in the face of an urgent, mysterious threat, it's the best conceivable way of limiting harm. Either way it's vitally important.

# 5. Information & Misinformation

*"To be charged with hubris is therefore an extremely serious matter, and not to be dealt with by murmuring things about antiscience and antiintellectualism, which is what many of us engaged in science tend to do these days."*[1]

So far, three core concepts have been deeply woven throughout these investigations: knowledge, honesty and trust. We've repeatedly witnessed the importance of candidly assessing our respective levels of knowledge—or the lack thereof—in both the scientific and political domains (and their overlap), and I've briefly touched on aspects of their complex and often problematic association with the notion of trust through the knee-jerk response, "Trust the Science!"

In this chapter the issue of trust gains center stage, as we move from the examination of public policy formation to the consideration of what our recent experiences have taught us about how best to communicate key information associated with such policies to the general public.

My own personal conclusions, the sentiments of an average guy with no prior biomedical knowledge living in an industrialized Western country with an internet connection who was suddenly forced to try to make sense of what the hell was going on around me, was that, on the whole, things were terribly done.

Most egregious, of course, were the catastrophically erroneous proclamations, from the Chinese government's early emphatic declaration

---

[1] "The Hazards of Science" in *The Medusa and the Snail*

that the virus was "Not Contagious Between People; It's Controllable and Preventable" so movingly described in Fang Fang's *Wuhan Diary*, to the World Health Organization's blatantly unsubstantiated early pronouncements that wearing masks does not impact viral transmission to American presidential declarations on, well, pretty much everything imaginable (ingesting bleach, the naturally salubrious impact of warm weather, hydroxychloroquine, you name it).

But beyond that was the nagging sense of essential questions continually unaddressed. News programs were filled with lively debates of how to successfully "flatten the curve" despite the fact that it was palpably obvious that we had no clear idea of who was actually infected and thus could have no real confidence in what the curves actually were. Virtually nobody was talking about the obviously game-changing role that large-scale asymptomaticity was playing in making COVID-19 infinitely more difficult to control than SARS or MERS that at least some health professionals on the ground were clearly aware of from the beginning[2], let alone any serious discussion of how, precisely, those potential global pandemics had been brought under control.

You hardly needed to be an epidemiologist to appreciate—indeed, there were times when it seemed that being one was downright counterproductive—that the only way transmission of the virus could be significantly arrested would be through the rapid development and deployment of effective testing devices so that we could clearly ascertain who was actually infected and take concrete measures to stop them spreading it further.

But no: the two obviously distinguishing features of this illness that clearly rendered it a particularly daunting challenge to come to grips with—asymptomaticity and possible reinfection, its evil, vaguely-related twin—lay consistently unmentioned for months. Instead we

---

[2] See, for example, the February 4, 2020 entry in Fang Fang's aforementioned *Wuhan Diary*, where a doctor friend casually informs her that "*Perhaps only 30 to 50 percent of the people infected will actually develop symptoms.*"

were regularly bombarded with tales of people mysteriously losing their sense of taste and smell, shown pictures of customers having their temperature taken before entering public places and repeatedly counseled on how we might be able to successfully distinguish between whether we had contracted COVID or just had an ordinary cold.

And whenever a story would surface that touched strongly on these key distinguishing features—like when we saw that dogs could be trained to detect COVID-19 with astounding accuracy amongst those who were oblivious to their own infection—it would quickly fade into the background, summarily grouped into the *Isn't that interesting?* news bin together with reports of cats playing the piano, instead of being promptly recognized as the possible window to vital mechanistic understanding that they so obviously were.

And then a few months later, when the Pfizer/BioNTech, Moderna and AstraZeneca vaccines were—justifiably—triumphantly rolled out, both the Chinese (Sinopharm) and Russian (Sputnik) vaccines that were simultaneously being injected into millions of people were, inexplicably, almost wholly ignored by the media (well, the media I consume at least, given that I don't live in either China or Russia—I'm guessing it would have been the other way around there). The tacit operating assumption seemed to be that such vaccines couldn't possibly work, or at least not work very well, because our governance systems were superior to theirs, thereby simultaneously demonstrating a profound ignorance of the inherently international nature of modern science, the logical independence of vaccine efficacy and political structures and even more worrying, the recognition that successfully addressing global problems necessarily involves globally coordinated solutions (of which much more later).

More generally still, as mentioned in chapter 1, were my high levels of personal frustration that, having suddenly been catapulted into a position where I was forced to regularly contemplate how my immune system was faring, there was precious little opportunity to learn what that actually meant. How does immunological memory actually work, and why are some diseases "remembered" better than others? How can I be so certain that we have the internal capacity to generate specific antibodies that can neutralize every possible pathogen? How does the immune response "know" when it's the appropriate moment to trigger a number of additional possible measures to stop an invading pathogen? What is the "control mechanism" for such a decision? What, exactly, does it mean for the immune system to be "deficient" or "compromised"? Which parts are typically damaged and with what implications?

It's not that I was expecting daily immunology tutorials during the nightly news (although that certainly would have been superior to being regularly confronted with increasingly confident "TV doctors" condescendingly assuring me that I couldn't catch COVID-19 from the internet), it's just that I constantly felt that I had no *context* whatsoever to understand what was happening and what might be done to stop it. Why didn't we have a cheap and reliable home saliva or blood test, say, to detect the virus? What was stopping us, exactly, from developing *that*?

It wasn't that I felt that I was being given downright false information, but rather that to all intents and purposes I wasn't getting any meaningful information at all. The president[3] made regular national TV appearances urging us to exhibit solidarity and increased consideration towards the weak and vulnerable in this time of crisis, albeit rather hyperbolically declaring at the outset that we were "at war." The nightly news was filled with authoritative-sounding epidemiologists teaching us about R-values and the aforementioned "TV doctors" patiently responding to medical questions without ever intimating that any answer lay beyond their grasp.

---

[3] The President of France, it should be specified, who, for all his faults, is clearly both sane and generally well-intentioned.

The whole thing seemed much more focused on calming people down rather than communicating anything of substance. *Don't worry*, was the all-too-obvious message, *We are in charge. Trust us.*

Now, one of the principal features of trust, as we all know, is that it has to be consistently earned. Breaking trust happens much faster, and is much easier to do, than building it. So when the glib facade inevitably began to crack—when it became clear that we didn't know nearly as much as was first implied, or that the situation was vastly more complex than had been claimed, or that some of our suppositions turned out to be just plain wrong—so did a good deal of the trust.

But the key question, of course, is, Trust in *what*, exactly?

A consistently-invoked theme of those I spoke with for this project was the crucial distinction between the notion of trust in any one scientific belief and trust in the overall scientific process itself: what we must resolutely put our trust in is not any particular claim, but the importance of consistently assessing all such claims to ensure their continued validity, unhesitatingly discarding them if they no longer appear convincing in the light of new evidence. We've seen this sort of thing before in chapter 3 with the lurking implication that "Trust the Science!" didn't mean that we should trust any specific declaration but rather have full confidence in the overall process that gave rise to it—and thus also, conceivably, might one day give rise to its eventual rejection.

Indeed, some even speculated hopefully that the very fact that people have been so intensely exposed to the toing and froing of "science in real time" through this pandemic might, when all is said and done, give them a greater appreciation of science, serving as a concrete corrective to the common misconception of science as the straightforward heaving of one incontrovertibly-established fact after another onto an ever-rising pile.

But I disagree. And so does Lorraine Daston, director emerita of the Max Planck Institute for the History of Science in Berlin.

> *"I think that confidence in science has suffered enormously during the pandemic for reasons that were entirely avoidable; and the main reason is that it seemed as if what was scientific truth today was scientific error tomorrow, so that people came to think of this as the same kind of weathervane opinion as the latest political dictum. And I think that represents a really fundamental misunderstanding about the processes of science and to some extent the status of scientific fact. Scientists have been complicit in this, but science journalists even more so. So that instead of presenting current scientific consensus as 'to the best of our knowledge,' it has been presented as if it were a Platonic or theological truth—an eternal truth."*

If you are presenting information as "Platonic truths" then you can hardly blame the public for interpreting it as such; and it seems distinctively duplicitous to later say, *"Well, you should naturally have understood what I said in terms of the tacitly implied confidence intervals that are part of the rigorous process of science that we should all unhesitatingly adhere to"* when you are suddenly forced to publicly recant any particular statement.

If you are keen to have people develop trust in the process of science—particularly those you know damn well will be more inclined to uncritically swallow your information precisely because they aren't intimately familiar with the scientific process—then you have to specify the degree of uncertainty in your claims at the outset.

Which is exactly why, as we saw in the last chapter, Alex Quintanilha is so justifiably proud of Portugal's decision to painstakingly build public trust by forthrightly declaring that *"there were some issues that we simply didn't know the answer to"* whenever circumstances dictated. Doing so must have required a considerably larger and more sophisticated communication effort at the beginning, and I'm sure there were times when those in charge were tempted to just stand up and do what everyone else was doing: announce public measures in the standard "Because I said so" style of authoritative declarations to placate a restive public desperate for concrete answers. But they resisted taking the easy way out. And in the end they managed to do much more than "build public trust" about the process of science, they built public understanding of the process of science.

This distinction, I think, is worth dwelling upon for a moment. All too often talking about "trust" conjures up images of being forced to choose between several unpalatable options in the hopes of navigating one's way towards the least unpleasant outcome. Revealingly, this is often best illustrated in a medical context: if I am forced to undergo knee surgery, say, I do my best to hunt around to find the best possible knee specialist in whom I can place my trust. Of course, I'd rather not have the surgery at all, but having no choice in the matter my only real option is to find the most qualified person available, close my eyes, and hope for the best.

But this is not the sort of thing that is going on when we talk about "building trust in the process of science." If you asked me what the weather will be tomorrow, I'd reach for my phone and look at the forecast. I wouldn't consult an astrologer or a medium or carefully observe how often my dog was scratching himself.

Now, you might say that I reach for my phone because I trust the weather report. Which is true, as far as it goes, insofar as I certainly wouldn't trust an astrologer (at least an astrologer with no access to the weather report).

But the reason for such trust, in striking contrast to my putative knee operation, is not because "I have to put my faith in someone," but rather because I have long become independently convinced that the report will be accurate and thus help me in my daily life, based as it is on a combination of our knowledge of basic meteorological processes, a wealth of real-time data, and highly sophisticated, ever-improving, computer models.

As it happens, I am old enough to remember a time when two of those key factors were much less developed than they are today, resulting in short-term weather forecasts that were correspondingly much less accurate and thus far less deserving of trust. Perhaps even more significantly, my level of confidence in current weather forecasts dies off significantly the further ahead I look. While my phone also unhesitatingly pronounces on what the weather will be like two weeks from now, in no way distinguishing its level of confidence from one day to the next, I don't trust those long-term predictions at all, knowing a little bit about the manifold instabilities in complex thermodynamic systems and our ability to predict them as I do.

So, do I "trust my phone" to give me accurate information about the weather? Well, yes and no. But more to the point, I feel that I have a good understanding of what lies behind its various pronouncements.

All very well and good, you might say, but it turns out that being caught in the grips of a global pandemic is a lot more like your example of having to undergo knee surgery than simply checking the weather report.

And so it unquestionably is. But the essential point is the same, I think. Indeed, under such pressing circumstances it is rendered even more significant: it's not about persuading people where to put their blind faith, or forcing them to undergo some abstruse, undesirable "educational" process that will allow them to show off how "scientific" they are, but rather to step up and proudly display the wondrous tools we've developed over the centuries to help us flourish in both good times and bad—tools that, by definition, are accessible to everyone.

And if you step away from all of that, if the first thing you do when a full-blown crisis hits is to say the equivalent of, "*Never mind all of that, just do what I say because I am an expert and know better,"* you are doing an egregious disservice to everything you claim to believe in, suddenly finding yourself confronting people like Charles Foster who are saying things like:

> *"Amongst scientists, we've seen lots of dogmatic pontification. We've seen the old "scientistic" model of science reasserting itself—that is, an idea of science as effectively a catechism rather than a skeptical method of approaching an investigation of what the world is really like."*

Charles, it is worth clarifying, is not the sort of fellow who can be airily dismissed as an uneducated, anti-scientific, anti-progressive type, given that he is highly educated, passionate about science and quite possibly the least reactionary type of person I have ever encountered.

That an internationally-acclaimed writer, University of Oxford law professor, medical ethicist, veterinary surgeon and much more (don't get me started about Charles; I'm convinced he's really five people) says such things should most definitely bring you up short and drill home to you that you've been going about things the wrong way.

In fact, that *alone* should do it. Forget about anything else I've said or am about to say. Any bombastic, declaratively-inclined, appeal-to-authority-loving biomedical researcher reading this book would be far better off putting it down right now and instead ruminate deeply on what on earth could have possibly possessed someone like Charles Foster to utter such sentiments.

But of course there are no such biomedical researchers reading this book. Instead, ironically, there is a real danger that such pronouncements (themselves hardly lacking in the bombast department, needless to say), might somehow blow back and impugn those few who are significantly helping the vital cause of public communication.

Which brings me to John Tregoning. John is an infectious diseases researcher at Imperial College London and the author of the comprehensive and engaging 2021 book *Infectious: Pathogens and How We Fight Them*, deliberately crafted to provide the general public with an accessible overview of essential pandemic-related information.

Neatly divided into two principal parts—what we currently know about infectious diseases ("Ologies: Investigating and understanding infectious disease") and what can be done about them ("Solutions: Preventing and curing infectious disease")—the book presents the layperson with an insightful, deeply relevant and at times disarmingly personal read—precisely the sort of thing, in short, that I've been insisting is lacking these days.

That didn't, of course, stop me from criticizing John during our recent encounters (rather than evidence of my obstreperousness, I naturally prefer to regard this as a sign of my dogged determination to critically engage on matters of substance). Images of Lewis Thomas dancing in my head, I gently upbraided him for not spending enough time highlighting what we *don't* know about the immune system.

There are a number of ways to respond to such an accusation launched at you during a podcast with an unknown interlocutor in the midst of an exhausting pandemic. You could coolly respond that, as the book was already some 350 pages long, attempting to also include the veritable infinitude of things we *didn't* know would irrevocably extend it to an unreasonable length and comprehensively dissuade anyone from actually reading it, which would resoundingly defeat the whole point of the venture. Or you could argue that, given the urgency of the moment and the palpable dearth of other such resources for the curious layperson, it was already nigh-on miraculous to have managed to have brought it out in any coherent way whatsoever in such a very short time frame. Or you could simply refuse to answer, regretfully announcing that you have an urgent call coming in and would therefore have to suddenly curtail the conversation. John, however, did none of those things.

> "I hadn't thought about it before, but now that I think about it — yes, in the way that we outwardly present things I think we do tend to talk about knowns rather than the unknowns. That's really interesting: I think there is probably a difference in the way we approach the way we present our information compared to some other scientists. It may also be related to the immediacy and the relevance. If I admit that we don't know about how black holes form, it's not going to impact how people behave during their trip to Tesco.
>
> "And in many ways I think that's a bad thing. We do need to be clear that science is messy. There isn't one science or one scientist—we all have different opinions.
>
> "It's really challenging, because there needs to be a core public health message which should be put across, which makes it very hard, then, to have other people say, 'Well, we're not quite sure about this or that.' Because as soon as you start publicly disagreeing, there will be a sense of 'Prominent Scientist X from Prominent University Y disagrees, so therefore I shouldn't wear my seatbelt' or 'It's OK if I start smoking' or whatever."

Three important conclusions, I think, are prompted by John's comments.

The first is one we've already seen several times in various different contexts: "science" is actually a many-splendored thing that encompasses a diverse range of activities under one name. Developing a rigorous understanding of what killed the dinosaurs, say, is not the same sort of thing as developing an antiviral vaccine or, even further away still, developing a well-reasoned judgment on whether or not it is a good idea to confine people to their homes during a particularly vigorous wave of a raging pandemic. There are commonalities in approach, of course—but then, as we've also seen, there are also commonalities in approach between cosmologists and historians or inorganic chemists and judges.

Within what's broadly recognized as "science," an obvious distinguishing feature is to what extent your work has the potential to directly impact people's lives. This can sometimes be confused with the common division of "basic" vs "applied," but while overlaps certainly exist, the two things are distinct. Trying to get a deeper understanding of the foundational mechanisms involved in genetic mutations, say, is unquestionably "basic research," while discovering which sort of lipid encasement works best to enable an mRNA vaccine to successfully deliver its information to the body's cells is self-evidently "applied," but both clearly have the potential to radically transform our lives in relatively short order. Discovering how black holes form, on the other hand, is a significantly different story, at least for the foreseeable future.

The second is that there are times—such as those we are living through now—when there's an urgent need to **do** something. As we've seen Alex Quintanilha eloquently phrase it, "*Politics requires action; it doesn't have the luxury of time.*" It's all very well and good for the likes of me to shake my finger at the dangers of "scientific authoritarianism" and hold forth on the importance of candidly admitting our collective ignorance in order to produce a well-informed populace that will ultimately embrace the scientific process, but many people, particularly in a crisis, aren't really interested in any of that: they just want to be told what to do, right now, in order to deal with the monster banging on their door.

The third point to take away from John's statement moves us in another direction entirely from the one we've been traveling in, but one that is a sadly unavoidable component of the topic of "information and misinformation," particularly these days.

Up until now, we've assumed that good faith exists on all sides. The scientific experts may be in error, or overconfident, or enjoy the sense of being authority figures far more than they should, but they nonetheless honestly believe that the course of action they are recommending is the correct one to take. The public, meanwhile, might be too uncritical, or too incurious, or simply too desperate, but they are nonetheless entering the "informational exchange" without any prior biases or convictions or agenda, simply looking for answers.

But that is not, unfortunately, an accurate description of what is going on today much of the time. Instead, the world appears to be strangely suffused with thundering, dangerously overconfident types fiercely wielding passionate, evidence-free, opinions that they are desperate to impose on anyone they can find. It is difficult to objectively assess how many people of this description can be found throughout contemporary society (since they are so much louder than everyone else they often appear to be more numerous than they really are), but it's safe to say that they can't be ignored, however much we might like to.

And when John talks about the importance of presenting "a core public health message," my sense is that this is what he is concerned about: the not-unreasonable fear that any public scientific disagreement naturally opens up a space for such exceptionally dogmatic types to promote their own agendas, deliberately clouding the air by fostering the patently misleading impression that no broad-based scientific consensus exists on anything and thus every conceivable view (including, consequently, their own) is just as valid as every other.

This is, I think, a real issue, and not limited to matters of public health (although that would certainly be bad enough). When I complained to Fyodor Kondrashov, professor of evolutionary genomics at the Institute of Science and Technology Austria, about the mysterious reticence of immunologists to candidly discuss our incomplete understanding of the immune system with me, his first reaction was to speculate that the white heat of the pandemic could well have exposed them to the sorts of concerns that evolutionary biologists have long had to grapple with: that any frank admission of ignorance of any specific issue was liable to be seized upon by some rabid anti-evolutionists as "proof" that the entire evolutionary framework must be discarded.

Worse still, such efforts are all too often strongly reinforced by the media's steadfast determination to "present two sides to every story," leading to the sorts of situations we are all too familiar with by now: where the views of the Chair of the Intergovernmental Panel on Climate Change representing the collective efforts of thousands of scientists over decades is "counterbalanced in the interests of fairness" by giving equal time to some cranky Texan ranting conspiratorially about how unconscionable it is that the conclusions of some isolated, dissenting study funded by a consortium of oil companies was not given the attention it so clearly deserved.

The charitable way to put the situation is that most members of the media, the vast majority of whom have no scientific experience to speak of, falsely assume that the notion of "scientific consensus" is fundamentally akin to "political consensus"—i.e. nothing more than a manifestation of tribal allegiance logically independent of any objective reality—and so necessarily requires the intervention of an "objective third party" such as themselves to present a truly balanced picture of the situation to the public.

The less charitable way to put it is that the media is overwhelmingly focused on doing whatever can be done to satisfy its own interests, even if that means grossly distorting reality, which usually just boils down to stirring up the greatest possible amount of controversy at all times.

Most people I spoke to were inclined to lean towards the less charitable side of things, with the common view being that the pandemic served as a particularly vivid illustration of the failure of most media outlets to responsibly alert the citizenry to essential information.

Philip Kitcher, for instance, John Dewey Professor Emeritus of Philosophy at Columbia University and a particularly thoughtful and well-established commentator on the intersection of science, democracy, public understanding and morality, looks at it this way:

> *"If I were a good historian, I could probably find some places in the dark past where people have been as badly misinformed as they've often been during the pandemic, but it is very tempting to say, 'In the late 20th century, news stopped being about giving people information—it stopped being people like Walter Cronkite saying 'And that's the way it is' and everybody believing him—and it became 'news for profit,' and 'news for entertainment.'*
>
> *"That was the beginning, and then the internet just blew it out of all proportion. And as a result we've got all sorts of people now believing very odd things about what's going on and misinformation flows like a sewer after an enormous storm: it's just a colossal danger to public health."*

At this point, our earlier, subtle distinctions between "trusting the facts" and "trusting the process" that so concerned us a few pages back begin to look like quaint trifles by comparison. Once we begin to suspect that the usual vehicles for disseminating information throughout society are vastly more concerned with their own perceived interests than in assessing and delivering the quality of that information, things begin to take on an air of the downright sinister.

And just when you thought matters couldn't get any worse, in comes social media, turning the "information landscape" ever more despairingly upside down. As University of Exeter philosopher John Dupré puts it:

> *"I think people sometimes think of themselves as customers of social media: that social media is providing them with a service—and forget that they aren't actually paying for it. If they thought a little bit more about why they aren't paying for*

> *it, they would come to realize what is surely the truth, which is that they are not customers, but the commodity. More specifically, information about them is the commodity and it's being paid for by the actual customers of social media."*

What, then, to do? If the prospect of transmitting trustworthy information during a health emergency is daunting enough when no personal agendas are in play, it seems virtually inconceivable in our present misinformation-riddled age where technology so dramatically enables a cacophony of personal ax-grinding from all directions.

Into this profoundly depressing picture steps Elizabeth Anderson, Max Shaye Professor of Public Philosophy at the University of Michigan, with a possible way forward. Which is hardly to say that she is not intimately aware of the severity of the problem:

> *"In the United States you can see that the pandemic has been used to sow distrust in society, particularly around the issue of vaccines and whether they're safe and effective. Conspiracy theories about 'the Deep State' and 'elites' have been used to divide Americans and suppress vaccine uptake, and that has led to one of the worst death rates on the globe, at least among the rich countries."*

From this recognition flows an understanding of both what not to do and, even more significantly, what should be done. In particular, there is no point in trying to wish away the fact that virtually every conceivable issue around us has somehow become deeply politicized. It is, of course, frankly absurd that we've reached a point where decisions on whether or not to wear a mask or take a vaccine should somehow be associated with which political party we support, but just recognizing the ridiculousness of the situation does nothing, in itself, to change things. Somehow, paradoxically, it has become "a political problem," and so—in the words of Alex Quintanilha—we need to both recognize that fact and then act. How, exactly?

There are those who maintain that the best way to proceed is by holding a public debate on the issues where representatives of different views can openly argue their positions. But Elizabeth disagrees, arguing that doing so isn't actually motivated by a desire to communicate information at all but is rather simply a form of theatrical posturing, a deliberate reinforcement of the inappropriately politicized division that brought us to our current desperate position in the first place.

> *"In order to move forward you don't have a debate, because debates have winners and losers; and a lot of the resentment is coming about because people feel that they've been put in a loser's position. That's why I think it's important to move over from debates to storytelling. If you want to understand how people process information it's through storytelling. You have to let people—across partisan, racial, educational and social divides—tell each other stories—their personal stories, their personal encounters, what they know in person. Not what they got from Fox News or CNN or The New York Times—but what they've experienced in their own lives. People have to speak from the heart, and then other people's hearts will open up, but first you have to show respect by listening carefully to other people's stories and responding to that."*

Telling stories, then: capitalizing on our unique linguistic capacities to indulge our fundamentally social nature. Now where have I heard that before? Welcome back, Dr. Thomas:

> *"We are compulsively, biologically, obsessively social. And we are the way we are because of language. Of all the acts of cooperative behavior to be observed*

*anywhere in nature, I can think of nothing to match, for the free exchange of assets and achievement of equity and balance in the trade, human language."*[4]

If you want to evaluate our attempts to communicate information, you could do worse than eventually turn to our innate capacity for language. In fact, when you think about it, it's pretty unavoidable.

---
[4] "Communication" in *The Fragile Species*

# 6. Research, Evolving

> *"I cannot guess at the things we will need to know from science to get through the time ahead, but I am willing to make one prediction about the method: we will not be able to call the shots in advance. We cannot say to ourselves, we need this or that sort of technology, therefore we should be doing this or that sort of science. It does not work that way."*[1]

I've spent considerable effort distinguishing between particular scientific results and the overall process, but it bears mentioning that this very process hardly occurs in a vacuum and is thus itself subject to external influences. It is not so much that the guiding operational principle of formulating rationally-justified conclusions through a rigorous interpretation of the evidence fluctuates (we hope), but rather that the sorts of questions we are keen to develop reliable answers to in the first place are often strongly influenced by our current circumstances.

In particular, when you suddenly find yourself in the midst of a life-altering global pandemic caused by a novel virus, it is reasonable to expect that some of that might rub off on your research program, particularly if your day-job is centered around modeling how viruses evade the human immune system, like Brian Hie.

I stumbled onto Brian's name during my attempts to develop some rough outline of the research landscape of computational viral evolution. As the cascade of SARS-CoV-2 variants began to methodically work

---
[1] "Making Science Work" in *Late Night Thoughts on Listening to Mahler's Ninth Symphony*

their way through the Greek alphabet with ever-increasing levels of transmissibility, I found myself wondering to what extent we might be able to harness modern computer power to predict not so much which variants were going to emerge—which seemed pretty unlikely for all sorts of reasons—but at least which types of possible variants would be best able to elude our vaccine-enhanced immune systems' efforts to neutralize them (so-called "viral escape") and thus would be most concerning.

I had anticipated being promptly enmeshed in an impenetrable world of thousands of technical papers after a basic google search, and was surprised to discover that only a few obviously relevant items came up. The most intriguing one was a paper in *Science* called "Learning the language of viral evolution and escape" by Brian Hie, Ellen Zhong, Bonnie Berger and Bryan Bryson, that presented results of a computer model of viral escape based upon a machine-learning algorithm originally developed for human natural language.

This was not only precisely the sort of thing I was looking for, it also, for good measure, made an intriguing connection between biological and linguistic evolution that struck me as precisely the sort of thing that would have strongly resonated with Lewis Thomas, who had written dozens of essays on etymology and the evolution of language.[2] Later I learned that this correspondence between the philological and biological worlds was quite a common one, strongly influencing the thought processes of many seminal evolutionary biologists, from Sewall Wright to John Maynard Smith—which, among other things, makes Thomas' aforementioned reflections on how the premedical curriculum should be "fixed" by formally eliminating it as a category and mandating that all students learn ancient Greek no longer seem quite so quixotic.

Several days after flipping through the *Science* article, I made contact with Brian. He turned out to be a delightfully engaging fellow with a passion for early modern lyric poetry (coincidence?) who had just

---

[2] See, for example, Thomas' book, *Et Cetera, Et Cetera: Notes of a Word-Watcher*

started a postdoctoral fellowship at the Stanford University School of Medicine after having completed his MIT PhD, the core ideas of which were encapsulated in the *Science* paper.

He graciously agreed to participate in both a detailed podcast conversation and a subsequent filming session, which pleased me no end. I was naturally curious to learn more about his research, but in truth my needs were more emotional than cerebral: after a long string of despondent discussions grimly calculating the exact velocity at which the United States of America was hurtling down the drain, I desperately hankered for some tangible evidence in the other direction.

Which he duly provided, excitedly describing how he and his colleagues nimbly incorporated the sudden appearance of SARS-CoV-2 into their research efforts.

> *"The original version of the paper was on influenza and HIV, and that went to a machine-learning conference. And then the pandemic hit and we began to get a ton of sequencing data for SARS-CoV-2, and the spike protein especially, and it reached the point where we all said, 'We need to try this on SARS-CoV-2.' It felt almost like an imperative—this was during the crazy part of the pandemic when nobody knew anything and the entire scientific community began scrambling to do whatever they could to study this virus.*

> *"So we got enough sequencing data; we trained the model but we didn't have any validation data. And right when I finished training the model, Bonnie Berger emailed me with this new paper that had just come out on escape mutants against Regeneron's cocktail of two monoclonal antibodies. It was really a real-time effort: as we were training the model, validation data was appearing. Later on some additional validation data on antibodies from Jesse Bloom's group*

> *also emerged, so at the end we were able to include SARS-CoV-2 into the project as well as part of the final version."*

For Brian, the opportunity to collect the rancid lemons of a suddenly appearing coronavirus raining on us and swiftly turn them into the lemonade of productive scientific research must have been particularly gratifying, neatly enabling him to help his research career and the world at the same time. And it couldn't have happened to a nicer guy.

But as John Tregoning recounts, many biomedical researchers have not been so fortunate.

> *"One of the biggest challenges is that it has further deepened inequalities in the field, particularly people with young families who really struggled to do their research in this time. And I think we may see holes in people's CVs, which will damage their ability to progress in the next few years. Some people have done very well out of it and others have had a very challenging time. So that's something that will need to be addressed."*

Another thing that definitely needs to be addressed is the question of research balance. It's hard to imagine something more profoundly disruptive to the international research community than a global pandemic, where so many scientists suddenly drop what they're doing and focus their attention on the same problem.

It goes without saying that such concentrated intensity will inevitably bring with it a wave of new discoveries and deeper levels of understanding that are impossible to imagine at present let alone predict. But there is, as always, a potentially concerning flip side to all of that. As John admits:

> *"I think there has been a slight risk of gravitational pull of a lot of biomedical research heading into a*

*single direction, into this one field of COVID. I think that has drawn resources and people away from other fields, which may be slightly damaging in the long run."*

One of the ironies of the pandemic, I was frequently told, is that, before 2020, coronavirus research was not considered to be particularly glamorous at all. On the whole it was viewed as a niche, not terribly interesting field, with the heavy investment of money and top people being directed towards topics like AIDS, with its infinitely more complex, diabolically shape-shifting virus and dramatically greater number of strains. That so many AIDS researchers have transformed their research program and found themselves suddenly immersed in the world of coronaviruses is itself a deeply unexpected development to say the very least, whose full consequences might take years to see.

This brings us sharply to the general question of how specific research avenues are decided upon in the first place—a topic that, in my experience, most people—including, significantly, most scientists—typically don't spend much time reflecting upon at all. The naive picture seems to be that, on the whole, it's fairly obvious to know which particular directions should be embarked upon: that there is a widespread consensus "in the air" of what sorts of matters are worth addressing and what are not.

But things are often vastly more subtle; and here, too, the pandemic—by offering up a strikingly different counterexample to usual practices—has thrown aspects of the overall process into sharper relief.

Before I continue, another obvious disclaimer is in order. There is a large and well-established group of people—historians, sociologists, economists, philosophers and more—who regularly engage in tackling these sorts of issues, duly offering up professional insights based upon a detailed appreciation of a wide range of established data and past precedents. None of that, clearly, applies to me in the slightest: I make no claim to possessing any sort of formal sociological expertise and any conclusions I've reached have been principally arrived at through my own anecdotally-driven experiences. But there are, I believe, two points in my favor that should counterbalance those limitations:

> 1. These personal experiences are highly unique and particularly relevant to the subject at hand, consisting of eight years of building and managing a scientific research institution from scratch followed by another decade candidly conversing with a wide range of academic experts on precisely these sorts of subjects.

> 2. This is my book. If you want other people's opinions, go read theirs.

With that out of the way, then, let me now unreservedly proffer my perspective. There are three principal factors affecting what sort of research topic somebody decides to work on:

1. Intellectual disposition

2. Community recognition

3. Money

Of course all three routinely overlap. To take one obvious example of many: given the obvious importance that status plays in all human interactions, many researchers invariably find themselves more "intellectually inclined" to tackle questions that the community has deemed to be important, which, in turn, is evidenced by the high levels of available funding.

But often things are much less straightforward. On occasion outstanding research questions unequivocally identified as "truly fundamental" have almost no funding associated with them, as the community has long concluded that, since so many great minds have unsuccessfully puzzled over them for so many years, the chance of an imminent breakthrough occurring from any new initiative will be vanishingly small.

Sometimes internal sociologies are so rigidly hierarchical that universally endorsed perceptions of "what should be done" can be transformed overnight when a new doyen installs himself (and yes: in such circumstances it is inevitably a "he"), complete with a radically revamped funding scheme.

And then there are times, such as the one we're currently living in, when external events have the power to temporarily produce a large-scale change in "intellectual disposition," with thousands of scientists spontaneously plunging in to do their part to help us navigate out of the crisis.

In short, the different, subtly nuanced combinations of these three factors are veritably endless. But in my estimation, by far the two most salient factors of this complex dynamic involve 1 and 3: individual predilections for basic or applied research and government funding mechanisms.

Not unlike, rather more famously, the search for a rigorously objective definition of pornography, the attempt to unequivocally distinguish between "basic" and "applied" research is notoriously difficult—indeed even more so in the world of biomedical science, where implied practical implications can almost always be found lurking behind even the most fundamental mechanistic inquiries (compare, say, the obvious "relevance" of any conceivable breakthrough in genetics with one in cosmology).

But despite all of that—and again rather like pornography, as it happens—that hardly means that nothing can be said about the matter. While there is much fuzziness involved in drawing any specific dividing lines, there can nonetheless be no doubt that, *en gros*, there is a real and substantial difference in mentality between those who are desperate to develop an effective solution to a specific problem and those who are struggling to comprehend the basic underlying mechanistic processes.

Both recognize the profound importance of breakthroughs of the second type, but for very different reasons. Those of a more applied persuasion naturally regard them as means to an end: a deeper understanding of mechanistic processes drastically increases the likelihood that we will be able to develop appropriate techniques to solve the problem at hand.

Those inclined to focus on trying to crack the mechanisms for their own sake, on the other hand, while hardly diminishing the importance of such "applications" (duly interpreted as inevitable manifestations of the "fundamental" nature of their discoveries), are simply driven by the desire to understand.

In keeping with the recent spate of carnal analogies I seem to have found myself invoking, here is Richard Feynman explaining the basic research motivations of theoretical physicists: *"Physics is like sex: sure, it may give some practical results, but that's not why we do it."*

Well, fine, some say: it might not be why you do it, but it's certainly why we should *fund* you to do it. After all, goes the thinking, scientific research is a publicly-funded activity; and, as such, its inherent value should be assessed in terms of what those funders—i.e. the general public through the proxy of government organizations—are convinced is in their direct interest. And by this measure, the fact that basic research sometimes produces important applications is definitely worth noting, but that's no proof that supporting it is the best way, let alone a necessary way, to do so. Maybe, on the whole, our money would be better spent by just investing in more explicitly applied research across the board?

This is hardly a new debate. As can be seen from this chapter's opening quotation, Lewis Thomas was a vigorous and unwavering supporter of the importance of a well-funded system of basic scientific research, consistently concerned that governments might not recognize its essential value for our future health and prosperity.

> *"We will have to rely, as we have in the past, on science in general, and on basic, undifferentiated science at that, for the new insights that will open up the new opportunities for technological development. Science is useful, indispensable sometimes, but whenever it moves forward it does so by producing a surprise; you cannot specify the surprise you'd like. Technology should be watched closely, monitored, criticized, even voted in or out by the electorate, but science itself must be given its head if we want it to work."*[3]

This sentiment resonates strongly with Patricia Churchland, UC President's Professor of Philosophy Emerita at UC San Diego. Long one of the world's most respected voices at the intriguing interface of neuroscience and philosophy, Pat is widely regarded as that rarest of all creatures: a rigorous, internationally-acclaimed scholar who is never in danger of taking herself too seriously. She is also, I knew from our previous Ideas Roadshow conversation[4], an astute observer of science policy, and thus an ideal person to pose the question that I'd been increasingly wondering about: Perhaps the staggering technological success of the COVID-19 vaccines might inadvertently produce some long-term *negative* consequences, leading governments to conclude that their future science funding policies should be disproportionately skewed towards applied research?

> *"I think it is a worry that, because so much of science has been really directed towards certain aspects of the pandemic, people will see science as essentially in the applied business and will forget about the importance of basic research. And of course they are both important.*

---

[3] "Making Science Work" in *Late Night Thoughts Listening to Mahler's Ninth Symphony*

[4] *Philosophy of Brain–A Conversation with Patricia Churchland*

"But the thing is that basic research, often without intending to have an application, will reveal something or turn out to have a discovery, that is hugely important for curing diseases, or addressing diseases or diagnosing diseases.

The applications are typically quite impossible to see from the vantage point of pure research, but unless we have that we're frequently unable to produce things that will have a practical effect."

In her own characteristically dynamic way, Pat energetically followed this up with a litany of compelling examples, from Marie Curie's single minded fascination with pitchblende that paved the way for a spectrum of key medical diagnostic technologies many decades later, to how a stubborn, seemingly perverse fixation on subtle differences between prairie voles and montane voles eventually led to a deep appreciation of the crucial roles that oxytocin and vasopressin play in the mammalian social world.

But the most telling instance came, perhaps unsurprisingly, from neuroscience, where she contrasted two American government policies explicitly designed to improve our understanding of the human brain and thereby develop practical solutions for brain-related diseases: an NIH-funded program in the 1990s called "The Decade of the Brain" and the Obama administration's BRAIN[5] initiative.

Both programs involved a spectrum of dedicated experts, but the funding mechanisms were crucially different. Since "The Decade of the Brain" was administered through NIH, most grant proposals involving new techniques or methods of analysis were not viewed as directly relevant to human health and consequently went unfunded. The subsequent BRAIN initiative, meanwhile, likely informed by this previous experience, took an emphatically different approach: concentrating instead on the development of techniques, tools and methods

---

[5] Brain Research through Advancing Innovative Neurotechnologies

that could directly unlock a deeper understanding of the brain's basic principles.

And the results, Pat enthused, were simply stunning, with a deeply enhanced understanding of fundamental neurological mechanisms occurring in staggeringly short order.

Revealing though that certainly was, I couldn't help wondering to what extent such lessons had been comprehensively learned, not just in the United States but more generally throughout an industrialized world increasingly beguiled by the prospect of a quick, directed scientific fix for whatever ailed them.

And so it was that after spending several hours leafing through the detailed OECD policy paper "What Future for Science, Technology and Innovation After COVID-19," I resolved to contact its lead author, Caroline Paunov, Senior Economist at Head of Secretariat for the OECD Working Party on Innovation and Technology Policy, to explore her views on a number of potential post-pandemic science policy issues, not least of which being the balance between pure and applied research.

When I spoke with Caroline some weeks later, she was quick to emphasize, as not nearly enough people have, that the remarkable triumph of mRNA vaccines—unquestionably the pandemic's most conspicuous scientific legacy—should be properly understood as the applied culmination of decades of painstaking basic research, rather than a one-off, directed effort: *"A striking illustration of how supporting research without a clearly defined final objective can nonetheless be of enormous value."*

That much I had already appreciated. But then she went on to point out that:

> *"The pandemic has also broadly demonstrated the importance of harnessing scientific approaches towards clearly identifiable societal concerns, most notably but*

> *by no means limited to, climate change. We're seeing increased numbers of people recognizing the need for science to be placed in the direct service of society."*

This came as something of a shock to me, because in my mind climate change was so obviously a scientific issue from tip to tail—initial diagnosis, required solutions, assessment of the likely efficacy of specific policies—that I couldn't quite wrap my head around the notion that there were people who might think otherwise.

I'm not at all questioning the claim—I'm sure that the data fully supports her conclusion that the pandemic has engendered an increased public awareness of the merits of scientific solutions to these sorts of public policy issues—but I can't help feeling profoundly bemused at the notion that any reasonable person ever needed to be convinced of such a thing at all, let alone by a global pandemic. What did they used to think back in those hazy, pre-"new normal" days of 2019? That magic crystals would save us? That we needed more Ufologists?

Some things are best not to think too deeply about, I told myself. Instead, I focused on my upcoming conversation with Fyodor Kondrashov, an evolutionary biologist I had encountered in an oddly roundabout way through some early epidemiological investigations.

On the whole, it must be admitted, the pandemic has done little to correct my initial gut feeling that epidemiology is no more genuinely scientific than economics, which is to say not at all. Indeed, the closer one looks, the greater the number of structural similarities appear between the two disciplines—from dubious initial conditions to dangerously simplified interactions to an eyebrow-raising overconfidence in their conclusions. Economists, goes the cutting epithet, have an unerring ability to successfully predict the past.

Personally, I've long found this too charitable: careful examination reveals that they don't seem to be able to do this either, as any clearly defined request to know what, exactly, caused the Great Depression will immediately reveal. And you will have an eerily similar experience when you ask an epidemiologist to tell you what, particularly, was responsible for the extent of the 1918–1919 Spanish flu epidemic, how exactly it ended, and why, precisely, several almost-global pandemics like SARS and MERS managed to be successfully nipped in the bud.

But still, it was important to try to keep abreast of things. Perhaps, given everything that was going on, an enormous amount of disciplinary progress was being made. So when a newly-published epidemiological study modeling the impact of both vaccination and "non-pharmaceutical interventions" on the production of vaccine-resistant strains began making some waves in mid-2021, I rolled up my intellectual sleeves and took a look.

Much to my surprise, the paper was lucid, thoroughly intelligible and decidedly non-grandiose. The basic thrust was that while, as everyone expected, high rates of vaccination would decrease the likelihood of vaccine-resistant strains emerging, relaxing non-pharmaceutical interventions (i.e. mask-wearing, social distancing and so forth) before any comprehensive vaccination campaign was concluded would increase it.

It all seemed quite impressive and thoughtful, with the only criticism I had being that any reasonable person would have concluded as much before running any such simulation in the first place. But given my predilection for lambasting epidemiologists for their dangerous tendency to indulge in unsubstantiated speculations, it seemed particularly churlish to be criticizing them for methodically demonstrating the obvious. Finally, it seemed, I had found an epidemiologist worth talking to.

Except further investigation revealed that the senior person behind the paper wasn't actually an epidemiologist at all. The principal author, Simon Rella, was a PhD student at IST Austria working under Fyodor Kondrashov, a specialist in evolutionary genomics who was officially listed as a co-author on the paper. A curious business.

So began my interaction with Fedya Kondrashov, one of the personal highlights of my entire *Pandemic Perspectives* experience. I will refer to some of Fedya's other insights later, but for the moment let me simply report his concerns of the possible impact of the pandemic on government funding—a view from the basic research front lines, as it were.

> *"We don't do enough basic research. Obviously I say this as somebody who does basic research. But there is a real issue—a lot of scientists talk about this—a push to get us to 'cure cancer' or solve the problem with antibiotic resistance or do this or that disease. Obviously there's great value in this sort of research—I don't think that all research should be basic—but the only way to do basic research properly is to have solid financial support for it so that those who do will know that they're not going to be out of a career in three years because they haven't cured some disease by that point.*
>
> *"And in that sense government investment in basic research is even more important than applied research, because—as we've seen with this pandemic—in some cases applied research can be done by companies who are endowed by other financial means. So I do worry that this trend to get more scientists to focus on applied matters will be strengthened by this pandemic even though—as everyone knows—you cannot have an applied science program without the basic one. But this is not in the hands of scientists, it is in the hands of the funders. Because the scientists will follow the money: we will do what the grants pay us to do. So how will the governments be impacted by this? I don't know. I hope that basic research will continue to be funded and continue to be valued, but I do worry; I worry about this impact."*

Before we leave the question of basic vs applied research and to what extent the pandemic might have shifted the balance, I feel compelled to wade into some deeper waters.

So far, all the comments defending the merits of basic research have been made, or at least can be straightforwardly interpreted, in an explicitly tactical way: The primary goal of the scientific enterprise is to develop tangible, life-enhancing products and the most efficient way to do so is by funding basic research on par with applied research.

This is not entirely wrong. But it is woefully incomplete. And I can't help but think that the very fact that nobody else feels inclined to forthrightly point this out is a deeply concerning sign in its own right.

Not that I'm not intimately familiar with the landscape. As the head of a philanthropically-launched basic research institute whose entire annual operating expenses were met by public funds, I spent years loudly proclaiming how investment in basic science is a necessary component of our future prosperity, trotting out timeworn tales of spectacularly useful serendipitous discoveries and invoking hackneyed metaphors of planting trees at every conceivable opportunity.

Most of the time it was all pretty manageable. But everyone has his limit, and what truly pushed me over the edge from "defensible but incomplete" into the downright unclean was the unholy conjunction of Einstein's general theory of relativity and global positioning systems.

For decades the general theory of relativity had no known practical application, but by the late 20th century GPS technology had reached a point where tiny gravitational time dilation effects between clocks on the ground and orbiting navigation satellites needed to be taken into account to ensure the maximum possible positional accuracy. And suddenly, "basic research advocates" had their poster boy, involving Albert Einstein no less.

This is truly stomach-churning stuff of the highest (lowest?) order, and only serves to highlight how profoundly misaligned our basic societal priorities have become. It is one thing to loudly sing the praises of mRNA vaccines or modern cataract surgery or the internet—all of which I will most happily do at the drop of a hat—but quite another entirely to imply, even to the tiniest possible degree, that Albert Einstein's theory of general relativity, to my mind the single greatest intellectual achievement in the entire history of humanity, could be somehow validated by the development of a gizmo that more efficiently guides us to the nearest Starbucks.

Doing so is nothing short of obscene, but that is where such arguments of the tactical efficacy of basic research inevitably lead us once we fully detach them from any official recognition of the profoundly elevating merit of understanding the natural world.

OK, end of sanctimonious digression. For the moment, anyway.[6]

Basic research advocates come in all shapes, sizes and levels of tolerance. Take Stephen Scherer, Chief of Research at the Toronto Hospital for Sick Children, who through no fault of his own has frequently found himself in the position of having to patiently wait for one of my passionate tirades to subside, but for some largely inexplicable reason keeps talking to me anyway. I think it's because I'm Canadian. By all accounts Stephen exhibits tolerance towards everyone, but he is also a strong patriot, so if you are a fellow Canadian his demeanor veers precipitously towards the saintly—needless to say, a character trait I have taken full advantage of over the years.

He is also a wonderful scientist, whose determined efforts to co-discover the widespread prevalence of genetic copy number variation significantly modified our understanding of genetic mutations writ large and consequently earned him a well-deserved spot in the

---

[6] A much more vivid and eloquent encapsulation of these sentiments occurs in Robert R. Wilson's 1969 congressional testimony in support of funding what later became Fermilab. When asked to what extent the new accelerator was connected to the security of the United States, he replied, "It has nothing to do directly with defending our country except to help make it worth defending." See history.fnal.gov/historical/people/wilson_testimony.html.

scientific pantheon. Indeed, our first conversation in early October of 2014 was a somewhat surreal affair as it came a week or so after he, Charles Lee and Michael Wigler had been prominently placed on Thomson Reuters' annual "Citation Laureates" list for Physiology or Medicine, widely regarded as a sort of unofficial "short list" for the Nobel Prize, duly prompting a storm of speculation from the Canadian media on the prospect of a "homegrown Nobel Laureate."

Stephen, customarily, downplayed the whole business, describing how just making the list was a tremendous honor, before laughingly predicting that the most significant thing that was likely to happen to him the following Monday in the wake of the upcoming Nobel Prize announcement involved the duct cleaners who were coming to his home for their annual visit.

These days, a sizable chunk of his time is devoted to designing the optimal environment for other scientists to create breakthroughs, yet another area that COVID-19 has significantly disrupted.

> *"I'm really interested in this question of the impact of the pandemic on scientific research. I come from a long tradition of combining cutting-edge laboratory work with professional collaboration and interaction; and we designed our research institute here at the Hospital for Sick Children under that model. The rule I was always taught from studying the great institutions around the world is that you hire the smartest people, support them, and then have the best coffee rooms to encourage them to discuss and share ideas so those "eureka moments" are more prone to spontaneously arise. And now we have at least half of our staff working from home, and we're communicating by Zoom and phone and so forth...so I really wonder what's going to happen."*

In fact, Stephen was astonished to discover that by some metrics scientific productivity at SickKids actually *increased* during the pandemic—another important pandemic-related sociocultural effect that we would do well to spend some time mulling over.

Meanwhile, the pandemic's impact on research and scholarship takes us well beyond the confines of the biomedical world, a point that arose frequently, from Ann-Sophie Barwich's ruminations on how algorithms affect social policy to Michael Gordin's hope for heightened attention on the science of older people:

> *"Given that the COVID-19 pandemic is substantially more damaging to the elderly, the frailty of elder health is very much a topic of concern. The rising load of Alzheimer's and Parkinson's cases as the population ages globally is something that should have made us aware of this before. I think that the pandemic has the potential of orienting people to think about that segment of the population, and I think that historians of science could have a role to play there."*

For historian of science Lorraine Daston, on the other hand, the impact of the pandemic went well beyond broad speculations of what could or should be done. In her case it was personal.

> *"The pandemic has catapulted me into the modern era, because it seemed to me that, when confronted with two crises of global dimensions—the SARS-CoV-2 pandemic and climate change—it wasn't the United Nations, it wasn't the G8, it wasn't any other international consortium of governments that diagnosed the problem and worked toward a solution: it was rather the very loose, never official, always precarious, international governance of science.*
>
> *"And I became very interested in how that international governance structure came about against all the odds, and how it is sustained, in the face of virulent nationalism and fierce competition amongst scientists. So*

*the pandemic **did** change the direction of my research; and I am now in the thick of trying to understand the first international scientific cooperations and scientific organizations of the late 19th and early 20th centuries."*

Like some mysterious interdisciplinary tag-team, Stephen Scherer seamlessly picked up on Lorraine's internationalist insight by detailing the scientific community's exceptionally rapid and unprecedentedly global response to the pandemic:

*"It was really striking to me how the scientific community came together really quickly, at least those working on genetic aspects of the pandemic. Here at SickKids Hospital we were involved in a national project across Canada where we were sequencing the genomes of 10,000 Canadians who were infected by Sars-CoV-2 and typically had a severe clinical outcome, and there were other projects going on in most of the major countries around the world. Within a year we were already combining data to do very highly powered large-scale genetic studies to look at the contribution of genetics to the susceptibility to the virus. At the same time the technology developed to sequence the viral genome itself—you've heard of all the different names, the different variants, from alpha to omicron now—I think there are over a million different viral sequences in a public database now and more than a hundred thousand genomes of hosts. We're all sharing this data around the world in very careful ways—they're all based on consented participants—but the sharing has happened really quickly, and we're starting to see a real impact. So I think this is going to be important for the pandemic itself, but also more generally in influencing how science will play out over the next decade or so."*

The essential role that international coordination plays in scientific progress has long been recognized by scientists and non-scientists alike. What is generally far less appreciated, however, is that international coordination is not only necessary to understanding the major problems we are facing, but also—even more critically—to meaningfully address them. Which brings us to the heart of our inquiries.

# 7. Necessarily Global

> *"The oxygen in the air is not placed there at random, any old way; it is maintained at precisely the optimal concentration for the place to be livable. A few percentage points more than the present level and the forests would burst into flames, a few less and most life would strangle. It is held there, constant, by feedback loops of information from the conjoined life of the planet. We are already pushing up the level of $CO_2$ by burning too much fuel and cutting too much forest, and the earth may be in for a climate catastrophe within the next century."*[1]

Perhaps the single strongest message a scientific training drills into you is that what *is* has nothing to do with the personal sentiments of you or anyone else on what *should be*. You might be delighted with the particular way chemical bonds form or it might drive you crazy, people can take to the streets and demonstrate for or against them as much as they want, but nature couldn't care less: bonds form the way they do completely independently of anyone's approval or disapproval. So if you want to make any real progress in understanding what's going on around you, the slightest consideration of how it makes people feel is simply a dangerously irrelevant distraction.

This is most definitely *not* the way it works in many other disciplines. If you want to figure out why one politician is more popular than another, or deduce why one literary work eventually became "canonical" while another seemingly equally thoughtful and well-written one was wholly ignored, it is typically essential to take into account the beliefs, desires, and fears of large numbers of people.

---

[1] "The Art and Craft of Memoir" in *The Fragile Species*

It is principally for this reason, I suspect, that many people tend to generally characterize scientific activity as "cold" and "unemotional," with all the consequent nonsensical biases about the "Spock-like" orientations of its practitioners that we saw earlier. This is, I think, a pretty odd way to look at things—and, if you step back and reflect upon it for a moment, deeply narcissistic.

After all, there is no reason to assume that the universe should behave in a conspicuously dolphin-pleasing or dog-pleasing way either; and if we want to comprehend bee behavior, for example, the sole conceivable way to do so is by adopting a distinctively bee-centered perspective of the world.

Which is all to say that the only time it makes sense to explicitly factor in human attitudes is when we want to understand human behavior in some particular way—which, self-absorbed creatures that we are, seems to happen quite frequently.

To invoke a scientific term, the general point to be made is that it is essential to recognize the appropriate domain of your problem in order to solve it.

To take an example of some contemporary relevance, if the problem is, *How the hell do we rid ourselves of this alarmingly megalomaniacal politician who is imperiling the very future of our country and significantly threatening global stability?* The answer must, logically, involve an attempt to penetrate the hearts and minds of the many deeply dissatisfied people who have mysteriously come to the conclusion that an important way to improve their lives is to elect this person to high office. Because that is the relevant domain.

Under such circumstances it makes absolutely no sense to declaim, "We need more democracy!" because the problem *arose* in the very context of a democratic system (more or less) and is therefore nothing less than a concrete manifestation of the beliefs and desires of those who were directly responsible for putting him into power in the first place.

Had the politician in question grabbed power through a military coup, say (which might well, of course, happen in the future), the relevant domain of the problem would properly shift to considering how best to ensure that democratic structures can protect themselves from armed threats.

And it is equally nonsensical to believe, as many seem to, that the full scope of the problem will promptly disappear if said politician gets hits by a truck or is somehow convinced to benignly live out his days in some remote Floridian *orangerie*. The notion that he is somehow the only possible person who could significantly tap into the aforementioned widespread dissatisfaction when there are obviously truckloads of others who would enthusiastically rush into any void caused by his absence is laugh-out-loud absurd, needlessly elevating a petty narcissist to the status of some sort of evil genius.

Even more misguided still is the conviction that the best way forward is to try to convince the supporters in question that their feelings and desires are wrong (or, worse still, that they are stupid), because that's so evidently not the way it works with human feelings and desires. A detailed study of the history of humanity will lead to precious little evidence to support the claim, "All we need to do is methodically show people that their beliefs and desires were wrong and they will change them."

I certainly don't pretend to know all the answers here, but one thought which immediately springs to mind is Elizabeth Anderson's recommendation that increased efforts should be made to explicitly create occasions for people to frankly communicate with each other. That suggestion, it seems to me, has the distinct advantage of lying conspicuously within the relevant domain of the problem and thus realistically represents a productive way forward.

You wouldn't think that you'd have to be a MacArthur Fellowship-winning professor of philosophy to come up with such a relatively straightforward idea, but clearly being one doesn't hurt your chances of doing so.

To summarize, then, the general claim is simply this: in order to coherently address any problem, we first have to identify its particular domain and then deliberately go about the business of constructing solutions that clearly lie within that domain. That is no guarantee of success, of course—there is a veritable infinitude of domain-appropriate measures that won't work—only that we can be quite certain that we are wasting our time if we've misdiagnosed the relevant domain of the problem and, consequently, that of the proposed solution.

And so, finally, back to the pandemic. The key insight here is that the domain of a global pandemic is necessarily international, which means that if we fail to explicitly take that into account any measures we invoke will simply not solve the problem to any appropriate degree.

As Duke University neuroscientist Miguel Nicolelis put it:

> *"Any military analyst would tell you that in a war in which you are facing a distributed enemy, you cannot face this enemy locally by yourself. You need allies. You need to establish a collective defense system through a global strategy. But we never had a collective defense system: each country decided to do whatever it wanted to do by itself; and each country created the optimal conditions, not for fighting the virus, but for fighting its own political and economic context. When we abandoned poor countries to their own local, minimal ways to fight this pandemic, we basically left open an open door—in military terms we got flanked by the virus: our right flank was totally exposed. That's what people don't understand: a virus that mutates in South Africa as we saw with omicron, in two weeks was capable of doubling the number of daily cases in Great Britain from 49,000 to more than 100,000 a day."*

We'll hear more from Miguel shortly, but for the moment let's turn to Gavin Yamey, Director of the Center for Policy Impact in Global Health at Duke University, for a disturbingly reinforcing message:

*"I was involved in some of the earliest discussions around how we could establish a system of sharing a vaccine, to set in place a system that would create incentives for countries to **not** hoard, to recognize that it would be better for **them**—the rich countries themselves—if all countries got vaccinated, not just the rich countries.*

*"And in the end what happened is that the rich countries behaved worse than even our very worst nightmares: they were more avaricious and more greedy and more self-centered, screaming "Me first! Me only!" in a way that really shook my faith in the idea that there really could be international health cooperation.*

*"I really wish that world leaders in rich nations had used their soapbox to explain to their citizens that it's in the citizens' interests to share doses.*

*"Now, I will go to my death bed believing that we should be vaccinating the world because it is the right thing to do, it is the moral thing to do: all lives are equal.*

*"But beyond that, there is **also** an enlightened self-interest in vaccinating the world; and we've seen this play out. We know that if you leave viral transmission uncontrolled anywhere in the world you increase the risk of new variants of concern. And we also know that it's economically terrible for rich countries when lower to middle income countries have awful outbreaks and aren't vaccinated; that's because supply chains get interrupted and trade gets interrupted and imports get interrupted."*

Gavin's explicit separation of moral and practical factors, together with a clear-eyed recognition of their conspicuous overlap in this case, is particularly significant. We all know that there are times when we are faced with a trade-off between general efficacy and appropriate moral behavior. Our understanding of fundamental neurological processes, say, would doubtless be much more rapidly enhanced if we would start conducting experiments directly on humans, but it is widely appreciated that in most cases doing so would be morally egregious. So we don't.

But in this case, it happily turns out that there is no need to worry about any of that sort of thing at all: doing the right thing turns out to be doing the very thing required to best address the problem. Which makes it doubly concerning when we don't do it.

We'll move to moral issues in the next chapter, but for the moment let's put all of that aside and simply return to our general, pragmatic, much-belabored argument that successfully dealing with any issue necessarily requires a recognition of its domain in order to construct appropriate solutions.

Both Miguel and Gavin emphasize the same two points: that the domain of this problem is undeniably international and thus necessarily requires an explicitly international response; and that up to now we've been sadly incapable of recognizing that basic fact and acting accordingly.

This might not matter so much if the pandemic could properly be viewed as a unique, one-off type of event—a sort of "100-year storm" in insurance parlance that was distinctly at odds with anything we'd experienced previously or were likely to experience in the future. True, our efforts to directly address it would largely fail, but pandemics will somehow end anyway—it's not like the 1918–19 flu epidemic ended as a result of comprehensive, internationally-coordinated, scientifically-enlightened actions.

In fact, that is precisely the way I used to look at the situation, a view that was subtly tied to my determination to launch the *Pandemic Perspectives Project* in the first place: something crazily unexpected, profoundly different and deeply unpleasant has happened to us, so let's at least take some time to harness the exceptional circumstances and extract something positive from the whole business before we rush back to our normal lives.

But that turns out to be a colossally wrong way to look at things, because on reflection the most significant thing about the pandemic doesn't actually have much to do with the pandemic at all. And intriguingly, many of the people I spoke with for this project had already figured this out long before I did.

Here, for example, is University of Michigan business professor Andy Hoffman's big-picture perspective:

> *"I look at COVID as a test of our institutions. Some held, some bent and some broke. It's a trial run for how we deal with climate change or species extinction or any globally important issue that requires the collective action of human beings around the earth."*

And here's John Dupré's conclusion:

> *"It's a rehearsal for the even more existential crisis of climate change, where we will have the same needs for behavioral change; and we're already seeing the same ability to ignore scientific fact because people's sources of information are just disconnected from truth."*

And here's John Dunn's summary:

> *"We don't know that any form of state yet realized is going to be adequate to prevent the world being completely*

*wrecked as a human habitat. And if it isn't, it only won't be because in fact the level of political performance in societies across the world improves sharply."*

Time after time, person after person, in filmed sessions, podcast conversations or informal discussions, the same message kept coming back to me: this isn't just a temporary health crisis; this is about our future.

The most penetrating analysis of all, so firmly in keeping with the thrust of this chapter, was made by Fedya Kondrashov.

> *"This pandemic highlights that we are truly, really, all in the same boat. Prior to this pandemic, many people approached their daily life with the mentality: 'My neighbor believes that the earth is flat, but it doesn't really impact me; who really cares?' And we were also used to countries having their own individual, local, solutions to problems.*
>
> *"But this pandemic highlighted that both attitudes are unsustainable: it is actually a problem if a lot of your neighbors believe that the earth is flat. Maybe not an immediate problem, but eventually it might become a problem. If those neighbors are refusing to wear a mask or vaccinate, this is an immediate problem. It is really an immediate problem when there is not enough vaccine equity in the distribution across countries. It's a problem if in affluent Western communities a large fraction of the population continue to refuse to vaccinate. So to me that was the most striking thing: as big as we think this world is, we're really all in this together. There aren't going to be 'local solutions' to the pandemic; it's not like this one particular continent or one particular country or one particular community could 'ride it out' while the rest of the world does something different.*

> *"Hopefully we will be able to learn from this and be able to apply what we've learned from this particular disaster and crisis to another upcoming disaster and crisis which is, of course, the climate-change crisis, because this is exactly the same sort of thing.*
>
> *"Having said that, I don't have any real idea how a genuinely integrated response between local and global can be made better. To me that is what is most surprising and fearful: that we seem to be incapable of having a united, scientifically-driven response to a truly global problem. We are completely screwing it up."*

For various reasons I decided to excise this last paragraph from the final edit of the film, but it is really the most chilling. It's not just that we've been extremely slow to recognize that we're now in a different and unfamiliar domain. And it's not just that, consequently, we haven't yet found a way to develop and implement appropriate solutions. The terrifying, yet undeniable, conclusion is that, so far at least, there's not one shred of evidence that we're *ever* going to get there. We're not making any progress at all. We are, in Fedya's depressingly acute phrase, "completely screwing it up."

Miguel Nicolelis, the charming and charismatic Brazilian neuroscientist who is the furthest thing imaginable from a wallowing, glass-half-empty, Eeyore-like figure, expressed it this way:

> *"We don't have a global business plan for the dialogue between scientists and politicians. This doesn't exist. Those types of meetings that occur for climate change are just all for show. We should have a global scientific committee with teeth, with power—not just pro forma. We should have a global scientific committee with subcommittees for all the major problems that humanity faces—and the planet faces—because it's not only human beings. We are losing bees in the*

> *billions. We are losing insects in the billions. And without insects, without birds, we'll die. We won't have anything to eat because they are essential to our crops. We are losing the ability to have clean water. The Amazon rainforest is going to be gone before I die. We have problems that are all global, and we only have local attitudes, or local initiatives."*

Aside altogether from the key "necessarily global" domain problem I have been focusing on, an added difficulty with "environmental issues" is that this very label is an emphatically wrong way to look at things.

"Environmental issues" should not be summarily dumped into some large public policy classification scheme like education reform or infrastructure development, not least of which because ensuring a healthy environment is clearly on a different footing as it is a necessary prerequisite for *any* aspect of human flourishing.

We don't have heated public debates (well, not yet, at any rate) on whether we should invest in better broadband or readily available clean drinking water, because it is understood that the former makes no sense without the latter. Most public policy issues involve a choice of some sort. Ensuring a healthy environment, meanwhile, is clearly on another level entirely: it is a necessity.

It goes without saying (but like a lot of things that go without saying, one is often forced to say it anyway) that things are considerably more complicated in the developing world. If you have to choose between polluting the environment and effectively condemning large numbers of your citizens to penury and death, then matters get drastically more complicated. But that is simply not the situation for those of us fortunate to live in the industrialized world.

So, one reason to reject the spurious categorization of "environmental issues" is that we are dealing with a substantially different priority level than almost any other area. But there is another salient reason, which is that the very act of separating out different policy sectors increases the likelihood that we will view them as independent from each other (such as my silly example of broadband vs clean drinking water). In reality, however, things are not like that, as Joanna Haigh, Emeritus Professor of atmospheric physics at Imperial College London, explains:

> *"It's not a zero-sum game. If you spend money on health issues, it doesn't necessarily mean that you're not addressing other issues. Quite the opposite: the best way of looking at these things is to address issues in parallel or symbiotically.*
>
> *"Many of the root causes of climate change also increase the risk or impact of pandemics. One simple example is that deforestation for agricultural purposes forces animals to migrate. And we know that when animals migrate they can take diseases and other things with them, pass them on to other animals; and, indeed, to humans. So, addressing the issue of deforestation can help the health issues.*
>
> *"In fact, it turns out that almost any action that you take on climate change has a positive effect on health. That's quite an interesting result."*

There is clearly a great deal of wisdom contained in all of this, but I was most struck by Jo's last words—*"That's quite an interesting result"*—which tacitly demonstrates a fundamental aspect of the scientific attitude that it is so clearly distinct from its political counterpart with which it is so often falsely conflated.

Because the clear implication she is making by stating things in this way is that the claim that, "Almost any action that you take on climate change has a positive effect on health," is neither self-evidently true nor one that couldn't have turned out to be falsified. That is, to return to my earlier point, it is not that we *want* the claim to be true that convinces us of its validity, or that it is a consequence of our advanced moral sensibilities, or that it follows naturally from the fact that many others also adhere to it, but simply that a careful analysis of the data happens to support it—thereby making it "quite an interesting result" in the classic British understated tradition.

Of course, the fact that it confirms our prior suspicions and resonates strongly with our personal beliefs makes us feel good, but that's not *why* we believe it. We believe it because there is sufficient evidence for it.

At this point I can well imagine you feeling somewhat perplexed by the decidedly disconsolate tone of my recent comments. OK, you might say, I'll grant you that this "domain problem" you keep going on about is both real and important: we now find ourselves in a situation where many of our pressing problems—including, but by no means limited to the pandemic—are global in nature and thus necessarily require a coherent, globally coordinated solution. And yes, it seems that so far we are off to a rocky start: we haven't yet developed any of the appropriate mechanisms to actually go about doing that. But isn't it way too early to be so despondent about it? Aren't you overreacting a bit?

Well, hopefully.

But to understand my concern better, let's turn back to Jo's insights[1]:

> *"The eye-watering amounts of money that have appeared, apparently from nowhere, in order to address the pandemic are quite…interesting. If something is prioritized, if we all focus our attention on doing something, then it can be done; and I'm sure that applies to climate change as much as to health issues."*

---

[1] Joanna Haigh is not only a highly respected atmospheric physicist, but was also the longtime Co-Director of Imperial College's Grantham Institute – Climate Change and the Environment.

What really worries me, in short, is not that our present and future challenges are too difficult to comprehend, or that they are somehow inherently intractable, or that the formal structures to address them don't currently exist. It is that, somehow, inexplicably, we simply don't seem to care very much.

In other words, it is a question of values.

# 8. Values

> *"We have an obligation to ensure something more like fairness and equity in human health. We do not have a choice, unless we plan to give up being human. The idea that all men and women are brothers and sisters is not a transient cultural notion, not a slogan to make us feel all warm and comfortable inside. It is a biological imperative."*[2]

A characteristic problem associated with any attempt to gauge societal values is that so much is constantly in flux that it is extremely difficult to say anything definitive about any prevailing beliefs at any time or place with any degree of confidence. How do we know when the change in attitudes towards legalizing marijuana or gay marriage or the abolition of the death penalty really began, or to what extent they have well and truly entered the hearts and minds of people even now? Well, we don't, of course. The best we can do is to try to piece things together and make educated guesses based on a disparate collection of potentially relevant information: the passing of related laws and policies, public opinion polls, the relative frequency of key words appearing in the media and so forth.

But one of the very few positive aspects of a global pandemic is that it offers a potentially more rigorous occasion to assess such matters. Trying to evaluate broad-based sentiments of global inequality between 2010 and 2015, say, is a vastly more nebulous sort of task than attempting to do so through the prism of vaccine-sharing during a pandemic, not just because the time period is (hopefully) relatively

---
[2] "Obligations" in *The Fragile Species*

short and well-defined, but also because there is a specific action—or inaction—to base one's judgment on. There is nothing like a genuine crisis, in other words, to illuminate the extent to which we actually believe what we've long maintained that we do.

And most of the people I talked to, you likely won't be surprised to discover by now, did not come to a glowingly positive conclusion.

A good place to begin is with Samuel Moyn, Henry R. Luce Professor of Jurisprudence at Yale University. I'd never spoken to Sam before our remote filming session, but it turned out to be one of those particularly gratifying situations where an author you've long admired is exactly what you've imagined him to be in person: measured, engaging and deeply insightful. Which, under the circumstances, made his comments even more troubling.

> *"I think that civilization is always on trial; and the pandemic has been a really high profile moment for judging the credibility of our collective ethics. Mahatma Gandhi, when asked what he thought of Western civilization, famously replied that it would be a good idea someday. I think that's true of us as a society and as a global community—glaringly so in response to the pandemic, when we realize that we have arrangements that allow mass death, and it really matters where you are on the globe as to how far you're exposed to it. We're at the beginning of learning morality and institutionalizing it, and I think the pandemic proves that one more time. It revealed an open secret to people who could have known but didn't and now do."*

Philip Kitcher, meanwhile, the often doggedly optimistic Columbia University philosopher we met in chapter 5, who has written at some length on the notions of ethical practice and moral progress, summed it up this way:

> *"By and large, I don't think that the reaction to the pandemic has shown us to be morally deep and thoughtful human beings. We haven't analyzed the moral situation at all clearly. We haven't recognized that the fundamental inequalities in our society are at the basis of certain kinds of reactions to policy making: that those who are struggling in our society find it difficult to take part in things that well-off people take for granted and recommend as ways of responding to the threat of infection. There have been all sorts of insensitivities that have been shown. Too little attention has been paid to the obligations of rich countries to make sure that people in the poorer parts of the world had access to treatments and preventative measures. But closer to home, we've often tended to demonize other people."*

And Philip was hardly the only person to notice how the pandemic greatly exacerbated such disturbing demonizing tendencies. It was also keenly noticed by Teofilo Ruiz—highly accomplished UCLA medievalist, legendary teacher, and one of the most genial people you are ever likely to come across—who naturally found himself looking to history to try to make some sense of what was going on around him.

> *"I have been struck through these last two years by the manner in which our response to the pandemic is pretty similar to the response of people in Florence in 1348. We have a great account of the plague in Boccaccio's Decameron, and the parallels between then and now are really haunting. One is that the people at the bottom suffer the most, which is certainly the case today in this country, where minorities have suffered more than others. There are also other parallels. In 1348 there was a widespread demonization of religious minorities who were accused of being responsible for the plague. This parallels some of the political discourse throughout the world, and specifically*

> *in this nation, in which immigrants and minorities have been accused of being conduits for the pandemic."*

Which brings me squarely to Teo's UCLA colleague Michael Berry, professor of modern Chinese literature and film and acclaimed literary translator, who offered some trenchant analysis of one such type of "demonizing political discourse."

> *"You would think that the virus would be completely unrelated to issues of trade and international competition, but it's actually become intimately intertwined with those precise issues. Initially, the US government actually applauded China's handling of what was happening in Wuhan. But very quickly, once it became clear that this was turning into a global pandemic, the political discourse changed radically, as politicians in Washington decided that they could gain some political clout from playing with it, leveraging it. That's when we start seeing the use of racist terms like 'China Virus,' 'Kung Flu,' and other disparaging ways in which the virus was racialized in terms of its associations with China or the Chinese people. And that, in turn, unleashed all kinds of violence against members of the Asian-American community and indeed Asians globally."*

Aside altogether from the transparently obvious point that demonizing minority groups is patently repugnant, these days there are additional tactical concerns that come into play. Because one of the conspicuous things to note about "minority groups" is that in other parts of the world they actually make up the majority, with all of the corresponding consequences. As Michael says:

> *"What a lot of people don't see, though, is once that politicization started to move into place, China responded in kind. If you're attuned to discourse on Chinese social media*

> *and Chinese mainstream media, you'll see that congruent to that is an incredibly visceral rise in anti-American sentiment."*

Contemporary problems of tribalism and xenophobia, in other words, are also—for better or worse—steadily undergoing a pivotal "domain shift" from local to global, a conclusion that certainly didn't escape the notice of the perspicacious Dartmouth College intellectual historian Darrin McMahon, a keen observer of the complex interaction of beliefs and social forces over broad stretches of time and place.

> *"You would think that the pandemic would force us to realize the obvious: that our problems today, our most pressing problems, are global in nature and that they demand global responses. Yet we've seen the continuation of intense nationalism. You would think that the pandemic would unite us in the face of a common enemy and we would come together to fight it. But in society after society, we see increasing social division."*

We've also seen a spectrum of potentially mitigating ethical measures *not* taken, despite the repeated urgings of many concerned and knowledgeable people, such as Richard Frank, Director of the USC-Brookings Schaeffer Initiative on Health Policy at Brookings Institution and Margaret T. Morris Professor of Health Economics at Harvard Medical School.

> *"The carnage that occurred in long-term care facilities in this country was deeply troubling: the slow response to protecting people who are in an environment where it was fairly clear that a disease like COVID-19 could spread very quickly. We didn't take the precautions and we didn't respond very quickly to ameliorating that. We had a series of tools available to us that could have dramatically reduced the destruction created by the pandemic: scientific and public*

> *health tools, but also economic tools. We were very slow to guarantee people incomes in the face of the pandemic; and as a result some wound up having to take risks because they felt their livelihoods were at stake. If we'd had a better financial support response, if we had moved quicker on the testing and actually been humble enough to use the WHO one, if we'd been more serious about getting people to wear masks, I think we would have dramatically reduced the casualties. And I think that history will indict us for that."*

The obvious question that this woeful parade of human iniquity prompts us to ask is simply, Why? Why did we so often avoid taking morally-appropriate actions that were not only much more in line with what we constantly tell ourselves we believe, but actually often turn out to be more effective in attaining the desired ends than their callous alternatives?

You'll likely be unsurprised to learn that, once again, I have no idea.

But Miguel Nicolelis has a theory.

Miguel's international scientific reputation was built on decades of pioneering research in neuroscience, most notably in brain-machine interfaces. All of that is unquestionably impressive, but doesn't, in itself, make him a fun person to talk to. What guarantees that is his unique combination of a lively sense of humor, delightful irreverence for authority and unquenchable desire to engage in all sorts of speculative and highly imaginative ideas. Anyone who has dipped into one of his books will know precisely what I am talking about here, but if you haven't yet done so the following will serve as a good introduction.

> *"As a species, the abstractions we've created out of our brains, our collective brains, have become much more important than tangible aspects of our survival. A lot of our problems come from the fact that things that came out of our*

> *heads—our ideologies, our economic systems, our views of what freedom means—have become more important, and more relevant, than concrete information about how we survive as a species. Life, human life, has been degraded below our abstractions, the biggest of which is money."*

But however much we might be reeling from the counterintuitive notion that our moral failings can be better understood through the window of neuroscience, it hardly follows that therein lies the way out of the morass; as Miguel is quick to point out that, on the whole, scientists behave no better than the rest of us.

> *"Scientists have to change their mindsets too, because right now all they think about is their next paper, their next grant. I heard reports of people trying to sneak into labs during the pandemic even though it was forbidden to get inside because 'Oh, I need to finish this project because my grant is due next month...'; meanwhile the whole planet was going up in smoke!*
>
> *"And I asked some of my friends, 'Why don't you drop everything and help us calculate models? You're a phenomenal modeler, why don't you join forces with us?' 'No, no,' they'd say, 'I have to do my little tiny project because I have to apply for this NIH grant...'*
>
> *"The entire system needs to be reviewed: peer review, the way we fund science, the way we misdirect so much creativity towards just getting more money. The pandemic exposed a row of fragilities of the kind of civilization that we created."*

For some people, wading into the murky waters of human motivations drives one to ruminate on how we might structurally leverage our inherent selfishness to successfully create large-scale human economic systems; which, in turn, leads inevitably to a detailed consideration of microeconomic theory.

This doesn't apply to me, however, principally because my entire life's experience has overwhelmingly convinced me that the only thing positive that can be said about microeconomic theory is its noteworthy combination of tenacity and PR skills that have somehow managed to persuade everyone of its ability to meaningfully interpret human events without the slightest shred of actual evidence to support such a grandiose claim.

It is not that I am opposed to capitalism, you understand, nor that I am insensitive to the enormous importance that economic prosperity plays in our individual and collective well-being, nor that I am oblivious to the hugely significant role that the business world, in all of its many manifestations, plays in procuring such prosperity (not least of which because, in many cases, "the business world" is simply "us").

Quite the contrary, in fact: all this talk of money had brought home to me that it was essential for me to become aware of to what extent, if at all, the pandemic had concretely affected the corporate sector. Were values now changing there too? And if so, how, exactly?

Well, if you want to get a clear sense of what is currently making waves in today's economic journals, then you'd be well-advised to talk to an economist. Given my aforementioned determination to get a sense of what was actually happening on planet earth, however, I naturally turned to Andy Hoffman.

Andy is a business professor at the University of Michigan. In fact, his official title is Holcim (US) Inc. Professor of Sustainable Enterprise, which in itself is a strong tipoff that he is not your average, run-of-the-mill sort of business prof. A consistently vocal proponent of the importance of twinning environmental sustainability with corporate profitability long before it was fashionable, Andy is also an award-winning author and a remarkably likable fellow who has a long and distinguished track record of amiably tolerating my spontaneous, invective-strewn rants that these days are increasingly leveled at his fellow Americans.

He is also, even more importantly, someone who actually knows what is happening on the ground: teaching and mentoring students, advising corporations and regularly interacting with a wide array of business, environmental, community and political leaders.

> *"I've thought a lot about the role that the corporate sector might play in helping us find solutions to complex global issues because I'm a business professor, obviously, but also because I'm a human being, and I look at the powerful institutions in our society and how they can help solve the great problems we face as a species.*
>
> *"I don't know if it's coincidental, but the level of attention in the corporate sector right now on climate change is something that I've never seen before. I've been teaching this for almost 30 years. I've never seen this level of attention to an environmental issue. I've never seen so many jobs, right now, for our students, with the word 'sustainability' in it. It is changing. And in many ways, to my mind, it's a recognition that corporations are shifting their focus—not all, but some—from just a Milton Friedman-type of idea that their sole purpose is to make money for the shareholder to recognizing that they have an important role to play in solving society's problems.*
>
> *"I see it happening more and more. Corporations are starting to say, 'What role do we have, as one of the most powerful institutions on earth, to solve climate change, solve income inequality, solve COVID?*
>
> *"The vaccine was a historic achievement; and it came out of the corporate sector, you can't deny that."*

Finally, some much-needed optimism. And there's more to come:

> "My students have a level of passion and an engagement to address these complex global issues that I've never seen before—a sense of purpose and meaning and mission. So while this generation is definitely being challenged and formed by current events, in many ways they're also energized to address them."

Only a few years ago, I would have regarded the notion of clinging desperately to the salvific potential of the current crop of business students as the starkest sign of futility, if not downright insanity.

That, too, it seems, is what a pandemic can do.

It was at this point that I began to suspect that I might be starting to lose some valuable objectivity, with the original goal of exploring how the pandemic might reveal intriguing aspects of our contemporary societal values having been insidiously replaced by, *What could I find that could possibly give me hope for the future?* What I needed, it seemed, was a good dose of cool, dispassionate, analysis to pinpoint any revealing subtlety and nuance that my all-too-emotional state of mind had rashly overlooked. Which made me immediately think of Martin Jay.

It is hard to imagine someone more fundamentally attuned to matters of subtlety and nuance than Martin, the Erhman Professor of European History Emeritus at UC Berkeley, who has made a career of calmly and thoughtfully sifting through complex, overlapping layers of meaning of a wide range of thinkers and subjects, producing seminal works on the Frankfurt School, the notion of experience, visual culture, the theory and practice of intellectual history and much more besides.

I first encountered Martin in the fall of 2014 for an Ideas Roadshow discussion that I later realized was typically Jayesque[3], in that it forced

---
[3] *Pants on Fire: On Lying in Politics–A Conversation with Martin Jay*

me to profoundly reexamine everything that I thought I already knew. This one was all about the topic of lying in politics, triggered by his book, *The Virtues of Mendacity*. It was one of those rare conversations that I wished would never end: ensconced in a comfortable chair listening to Martin seamlessly weave together a diverse array of compelling insights from ancient Greek theater to Kant to Hannah Arendt into one somehow suddenly self-evident whole. We began, if memory serves, talking about baseball. There is nobody quite like Martin.

Of course, I knew it would take some doing to get him to participate, that his first reaction would undoubtedly be something along the lines of, "That's very nice, Howard, but I'm afraid I'm not the slightest bit expert in this area and so will have to demur."

Which was why I decided to start my introductory email to him by proleptically writing, "I'm certain that your first reaction is to say that you are not sufficiently expert in this topic, but please allow me to explain why I think that is not an appropriate response under these particular circumstances…," before going on to argue that, since the whole point was to simply record a wide variety of different views and interpretations of a specific, transformative event, there was simply no way, by definition, that anyone involved could be said to have any objective measure of "expertise."

Happily it worked, with Martin informing me that I had managed to "successfully disarm" his immediate response. Behold the degree of meticulously calculated preparation that is required to deal with the likes of Martin Jay.

But it was definitely worth it, because sure enough, once recording began, he promptly pointed out an intriguing value-related subtlety associated with the pandemic that nobody else had mentioned.

> *"In this particular crisis, what we discovered was an unexpected conflict between scientific expertise on the one hand and what we might call liberal human rights or*

> *libertarian human rights on the other, as there were those who argued that they had certain freedoms, certain human rights, that were being abrogated by a collective decision informed by scientific expertise. They argued that their bodies were inviolable, that they had a kind of possessive control over their bodies, and that as a result they would not accept the mandate of the government led by scientists to get vaccinated because this was an intrusion on their personal freedom.*
>
> *"Now this is a very complex issue, and we certainly feel in many cases that the body is indeed inviolable. So, as a result we are in a kind of crisis because of the conflict between two values that we hold dear: the idea of solidarity, public good and collective wisdom on the one hand, and the inviolability of the individual on the other.*
>
> *"Our society in particular is a place where this battle has been staged over the years in many different ways. We don't always come out on the same side; that's why the abortion issue is so extraordinarily vexed and that's why one has a certain, let's say, grudging respect for the position of those who feel that their bodies ought not to be intruded upon by the state. It's a complicated issue with no single answer, but we've learned a lot about the complexities of it as a result of how we've had to deal with the crisis."*

You see what I mean? This is a strikingly different sort of reaction than those many militants on both "the left" and "the right" who are too busy dogmatically trumpeting their convictions to notice that they might fundamentally clash with other ones that they equally vehemently maintain.

That's not to say, of course, that it is impossible to coherently believe in both a woman's right to abortion and the merits of vaccine mandates under certain circumstances, say, only that a deeper appreciation of the structural nuances of each position invariably yields both a better awareness of the depth of the moral issues involved and, consequently, an increased understanding of the opposing position.

To return to Elizabeth Anderson's point that we need to make a deliberate effort to listen to each other's stories, we can add that there is a greater likelihood that such a mutual storytelling exercise will be effective if we enter into the process with a deliberately elevated level of open-mindedness and tolerance.

Such sentiments are often invoked with an unthinking patina of condescension—*Look at how tolerant and open-minded I am because I am willing to sit down and talk with someone who is so obviously deluded!*—but actual tolerance, of course, flows from a sense of genuine empathy, which flows from a recognition that your opponent's position is in some ways defensible, which in turn flows from an awareness that your own position is not exactly iron-clad.

We all like to think that we're tolerant and that our adversaries are not, but the bitter truth is that we often don't go to anywhere near the lengths we should to forthrightly examine our own assumptions and biases.

In fact, the real problem is actually considerably worse than that: it's not just that our perceptions of how tolerant we are often don't match up terribly well with reality, it's that we have an alarming capacity for self-deception across the board, a conclusion that Charles Foster believes our pandemic experiences all-too-vividly illustrate.

> "Looking back on this period, historians of the future will be amazed at how fragile we are, how vulnerable we are, how gullible we are. We're not, we now know humiliatingly, the sorts of creatures that all our politics and all our sociology and all our economics has assumed that we are."

On reflection, then, perhaps the most salient thing the pandemic has taught us is not so much that we really believe X when we say we believe Y, but that we haven't yet carefully thought through what we believe at all.

As Charles concludes:

> *"We need to begin our political and sociological journey with an evaluation of that most fundamental question: What sort of creatures are we?—taking into account the lessons which have been so painfully learned over the last couple of years."*

## 9. Biology, Better

> *"The only solid piece of scientific truth about which I feel totally confident is that we are profoundly ignorant about nature. Indeed, I regard this as the major discovery of the past hundred years of biology."*[1]

A biologist friend of mine once earnestly told me that the single most terrifying phrase in the English language is, "I'm a physicist and I'm here to help."

Having managed a theoretical physics institute for the better part of a decade, it's not difficult to imagine what he meant; and many's the time I have reflected soberly on what it must be like for professional biologists to experience obnoxiously overconfident physicists strut into their laboratories and condescendingly inform them of how they must promptly restructure their entire working lives from scratch. This image, never very far from my mind during the writing of these essays, comes into particularly sharp focus during this chapter when I flirt dangerously close to doing precisely that. But still.

The vivid contrast between the worlds of physics and biology begins very early—at high school, if not earlier—where those who exhibit strong mathematical abilities and a predilection for formal thinking are encouraged to direct their energies towards Einsteinian notions of "uncovering the secrets of the universe," while those who exhibit curiosity about the living world are correspondingly steered towards a

---
[1] "The Hazards of Science" in *The Medusa and the Snail*

course of study that culminates in two of the most unpalatable human activities imaginable: rote memorization and dissecting frogs.

This is all wrong in far too many ways to count, with the unfortunate result of an undeniable undercurrent running through the scientific world that, when you get right down to it, physicists are just plain smarter than biologists; and that, should they somehow wish to, they could easily sort out all the issues their benighted biological colleagues are struggling with, but busy as they are with grappling with the pressing conundrums of dark matter, dark energy, quantum gravity and all of that (i.e. "secrets of the universe"), they really can't spare the time.

My principal concern, as it happens, is not so much the natural irritation this entails for biologists—physicists are well-known to be deeply unlikable people, after all, with their steady determination to make rigid judgments of intellectual merit rippling, fractal-like, throughout the entire scientific world, most definitely including sub-disciplines of physics as well[2]—but that such an outlook has insidiously penetrated the subconsciousness of the biological community itself, resulting in a deep-seated insecurity of nothing less than Freudian significance (see "physics envy").

This matters, I think, in three distinct ways:

First, there is the disproportionately large tendency of those in the biological sciences to embrace authority. I am certainly not saying that biologists are the only types—scientific or otherwise—to regularly invoke appeals to authority; and given the enormous breadth of "the biological world," a great many shades of gray exist, with the rule clearly being that the closer one moves towards medicine, the worse the problem clearly becomes, as I shall shortly touch upon. But still

---

[2] It bears mentioning for completeness that mathematicians generally sneer at physicists for very similar reasons to why physicists sneer at others—that they typically have an insufficient mathematical understanding—but since most people, on the whole, tend not to listen to mathematicians, this point is not widely appreciated.

and all, it seems transparently evident to me that biology is by far the most authority-riddled scientific discipline there is, a trait which seems inherently enmeshed in the biological psyche.

One obvious example is the Nobel Prize. It is hardly a secret that the Nobel Prize invariably brings out the worst sort of behavior among scientists, with a tremendous amount of behind-the-scenes scheming, post-award crowing and subsequent community-wide boot-licking. Pretty well all scientific prizes have these sorts of deeply unsavory aspects associated with them[3], so you would naturally expect that the biggest prize of them all would be the worst; and it typically is. But while many's the time I've been repelled by this sort of childishness in other scientific disciplines, it is nothing compared to the constant stream of Nobel Prize-related rhetoric that unhesitatingly spews forth from the mouths of almost all biologists. These guys simply won't ever shut up about the Nobel Prize for Physiology or Medicine (which should really make up its mind, incidentally): from trumpeting the value of a current result ("Nobel Prize-worthy") to diminishing the value of a current result ("hardly Nobel Prize-worthy") to—by far the worst of all—implying that a result can't possibly be reconsidered or re-examined in any way because, after all, "It won a Nobel Prize."

If you parachuted down from a distant planet and listened to a bunch of biologists talking for any length of time you'd likely conclude that the main point of their enterprise was to win Nobel Prizes rather than simply figuring stuff out. And—to return to our theme—in my more psychoanalytical moments, I can't help but think that all of this Prize-worshiping, authority-loving nonsense is somehow tied to a collective form of intellectual insecurity that has its roots in being universally regarded as the awkward, plodding, formaldehyde-reeking scientific sibling.

---

[3] For an innovative treatment of this "prize problem," the reader is directed to the insightful remarks of the exception-who-proves-the-rule foundational physicist Paul Steinhardt, detailed in chapter 1 of *Inflated Expectations: A Cosmological Tale–A Conversation with Paul Steinhardt.*

If that were the only consequence, it would simply be annoying. But in my estimation the major problem with this misperception of biology as somehow intellectually inferior to other branches of science is that it leads to a diminishment of the fundamental importance of theoretical approaches. It's almost as if the collective response is something like, *"Fine; we can't write fancy equations. But we more than make up for that by actually getting our hands dirty doing a wide array of deeply impressive experiments with beautiful, cutting-edge equipment."*

Now, I am in no way denying the overwhelming importance of experiment or the obvious fact that, due to its staggering complexity (a point that will be stressed shortly), the biological world naturally requires vastly more empirical effort than any other scientific discipline. But the concern is that, all too often, the field broadly defines itself and its practitioners as somehow *necessarily* empirical, which is, I think, deeply short-sighted and just plain wrong. Real biologists, seems to go the thinking, do real biology: they go into their real labs (which are funded with real money) and collect real data so as to find out what is really happening in the real world (in the hopes of winning a real Nobel Prize).

Well, OK. But we should know by now that "the real world" is often a lot less transparently intelligible than what we used to think it was, from the nature of a particle to how our brains interpret—indeed, pro-actively select—the information "the real world" is presenting to us. Which means that in order to make genuine progress in our understanding we not only have to get a lot more experimental input, we also have to spend a lot more time thinking about what such data actually means.

As Fedya Kondrashov poignantly lamented during our recent podcast conversation:

> *"It's a different thing in biology to have ideas and to have data; and data beats ideas in biology time and time again.*

> *When you asked me about what frustrates me the most about the current state of biology, this is it: that money and data always tend to beat ideas in our field. Because by spending more you can observe things on a different scale, but conceptually it's not necessarily anything different."*

Which brings me to my third point: a sure-fire way of perpetuating the status quo that so often disparages the very notion of "theoretical biology" is by ensuring that anyone who might be the slightest bit inclined to take a more formal, abstract, mechanistic, principle-driven approach to things is promptly driven into other domains, such as physics, both to satisfy her inherent intellectual orientation and avoid subjecting herself to mind-numbing memorization of the various parts of dead animals that she would otherwise be forced to cut into.

This dreadful situation is, thankfully, slowly changing, but not because of any conscious effort on the part of educators or leading (Nobel Prize-bearing!) members of the biological community, but rather because the benevolent combination of an explosion in computational possibilities and rapidly developing genetic understanding have given rise to increasing opportunities for transformative change through the unavoidable recognition of the importance of manipulating biological information.

But as gratifying as this is to see—and it most certainly is—I can't help but wonder how many thousands of intellectually agile and passionately curious young people are being driven out of biology at this very moment due to the thoughtlessly perpetuated, blatantly false stereotype that it is not the sort of thing for them. Sure, a few might eventually return via computer science or applied mathematics or even physics, but on the whole isn't this a terribly inefficient way to be doing things?

It is not, to invoke Joanna Haigh's description a couple of chapters ago, a zero sum game: I am not in the slightest way suggesting that biology should become "less empirical" in its approaches, only that it make a conscious effort to significantly broaden its intellectual horizons so as to involve vastly more bright young people in its research effort and thereby dramatically enhance its rate of forward progress.

Moreover, to explicitly reconnect with a point made in chapter 6, usually when people say these sorts of things, the tacit underlying motivation is one of direct societal benefit: we would have better drugs, or cure more diseases or develop more concrete techniques to address climate change if a correspondingly greater number of young people would plunge into the world of scientific research. That is both resoundingly true and unequivocally desirable. But it is not all.

In just the same way that I am incensed by the implication that a GPS device incorporating Einstein's general theory of relativity should in any way be seen as a reason to heighten our appreciation of one of humanity's greatest achievements, the notion that the only, or principal, benefit to meaningfully shedding light on the many mysteries of the biological world is encapsulated in a more effective pill is profoundly disturbing to me, roughly equivalent to evaluating Shakespeare's worth by his tangible impact on the pulp and paper industry over the centuries. It is a deep debasement of the glorious potential of *Homo sapiens*. It is not often that I sing the praises of my species (as you might have noticed), but there it is: dig deep enough and there is a rippling vein of pride running through us all.

So, what to do? What concrete, practical measures might we take so as to increase, even by a little bit, the likelihood of biology living up to its magnificent potential?

Well, we've already raised one obvious but important point: stop explicitly structuring your educational system so as to perversely drive away future contributors. To which we can add Lewis Thomas' incisive recommendation in chapter 2 that we should focus our attention on simply intriguing beginning students by highlighting what *isn't* known rather than forcing them to unthinkingly regurgitate what is.

And before we go much further, it's worth emphasizing that what we are talking about here is biological research as opposed to "medicine." Indeed, the elephant in our biological room that the pandemic has played no small part in further obscuring is the profound difference in attitudes between medicine and biology, with the former typically involving a degree of rampaging, unreflective pragmatism that would make your average mechanical engineer blush (which is saying something). That medicine is broadly seen by many outsiders as essentially "scientific" in outlook is yet another distracting irony of our current situation; and it's safe to say that if these guys are somehow put in charge things will only get worse.

I have no idea to what degree Lewis Thomas was an outlier in the medical establishment of his day, but what cannot be denied is that, eminent physician, hospital administrator and med school Dean that he was, he was constantly urging his colleagues to be on guard against overconfidence, while providing them with a litany of examples of how medical progress is deeply dependent on an independent basic research culture that must, among other things, dispassionately evaluate the successes and failures of medicine itself.[4]

The attitudinal gulf between medicine and biological research, I think, is not so much the product of the fundamentally different innate tendencies of its participants as the inevitable result of powerful structural forces that anyone who embarks on a medical career is unceasingly subjected to.[5]

From the first years of university (suffice it to say that Thomas' recommendations on "how to fix the pre-medical curriculum" we saw back

---

[4] See, to take one of many examples, "Medical Lessons from History" in *The Medusa and the Snail*

[5] I'm going to be very hard on the medical profession in what follows, but it's worth bearing in mind that my criticism is directed towards my perception of their general lack of scientific rigor, not their moral outlook; most doctors I have encountered are very decent people, and particularly so in France, which has a striking percentage of simply wonderful people practicing medicine.

in chapter 3 have not been widely implemented) to medical school—chalk-full as it is with struttingly hierarchical, sleep-depriving practices that extensive biological research has firmly established as blatantly injurious to human health—to an academic system where the salaries of medical school faculty are often exclusively met through their grants, the entire system is focused disproportionately on status, authority, money and immediate results.[6]

Anyone with a scintilla of curiosity or tendency towards impartial self-analysis will promptly have it beaten out of him after a few weeks. It is hard to imagine anything remotely "scientific," even by the broadest sort of definition, coming out of such a system; and it doesn't.

Any research biologist is naturally aware of the deep fault lines between her field and "medicine," but the rest of us typically aren't. In my case, the distinction was brought to a head, as it were, by my personal experiences several years ago when I was diagnosed with a benign brain tumor called a vestibular schwannoma. I say "benign" to distinguish it from its vastly more dangerous metastasizing relative, but the thing is, a steadily advancing growth in your head increasingly pushing other well-placed things out of the way is most definitely a cause for concern: something must be done about it.

So I tried to figure out what to do. The doctors in my immediate area had unhesitatingly recommended an invasive surgical procedure pioneered in the 1950s that involved severing the relevant nerve and excising the tumor, but a quick trip to the internet revealed that there was, in fact, an alternative: radiosurgery. There was, it seemed, considerable debate in the medical community as to which treatment was to be recommended, so I rolled up my metaphorical sleeves and

---

[6] See Thomas' customarily revealing remarks in "The Governance of a University" in *The Youngest Science*: "*I have lived most of my professional life in one medical school after another, and have a deep affection and admiration for these institutions, but I can see that some things are wrong with them and are beginning to go wronger still. If I were the president of a major university I would not want to take on a medical school, and if it already had one, I would be lying awake nights trying to figure out ways to get rid of it.*"

downloaded as many studies comparing the two procedures as I could find (the phrase "doing your own research," incidentally, carries with it very different semantic hues in different contexts: when referring to a determination to demonstrate the conspiratorial dangers of an obviously effective vaccine it is clearly a sign of some sort of mental turbulence; when used to investigate which deeply unpalatable medical option you should choose to best protect your quality of life, there is a strong argument that *not* doing so is a sign of some sort of issue).

All of this produced two striking conclusions highly relevant to the matter at hand (lest you think I was just seizing the moment to regale you with my own dismaying medical experience):

All the data pointed in one overwhelming direction: towards radiosurgery. And by all the data, I really mean **all** the data. I couldn't find one study that provided any justification whatsoever for the older approach even being on the table, let alone taken seriously. This I hadn't expected at all. Surely, I thought to myself, the very fact that there were two options implied that there were strengths and weaknesses to both, that both were to be somehow weighed against each other and specific circumstances taken into account? But no. This was simply shocking, even more so when you learn that the mortality rate for the older procedure was estimated at 1% as opposed to the 0% risk of radiosurgery. Now, 1% might not sound like a lot, but when applied to one's chances of leaving the operating room alive, it suddenly seems rather significant indeed[7].

So, who on earth would possibly recommend a highly-invasive medical procedure with a 1% mortality rate that a preponderance of evidence indicates is vastly less effective than a drastically less invasive solution with a 0% mortality rate? Well, one is forced to conclude, those who are already "invested" in such a procedure—those who had spent decades

---

[7] Put another way, if your chances of winning a lottery were 1%, you would be well-advised to drop everything you were doing and spend your time buying as many tickets as you could.

perfecting their highly specialist brain-surgical techniques. Which is in itself very impressive as far as it goes, but not terribly in keeping with my understanding of the Hippocratic Oath, nor, to return to the topic in question, remotely "scientific." So that's the first point.

The second point is, I think, perhaps even more revealing still: whenever I told this tale to my biological friends and acquaintances—neuroscientists, evolutionary biologists, cell and molecular biologists—none of them was the slightest bit surprised. In fact, a typical reaction would be a shake of the head followed by a sudden launch into their own similar anecdotes of flagrant medical unscientificness that they had encountered in a wide variety of personal circumstances.

Which is all to say that whatever one might want to say about the lack of sufficient conceptual rigor often exhibited throughout the world of biological research (and I am far from done yet), it is a horse of a very different color indeed from the sort of thing that one constantly encounters in its gargantuan, financially-ravenous, often-bombastic medical brother with whom it is so often confusingly conflated.

End of medical digression. It wasn't pleasant, but it had to be done, I think—a sort of intellectual triage before moving on to focusing attention on the core problem at hand—which is, you may recall, imagining how biological research might better improve. "Better improve" because—in striking contrast to contemporary theoretical physics, as it happens—it is manifestly obvious that biology will make enormous strides in the decades to come anyway. We are on the threshold of spectacular advances in our biological understanding, and all I am recommending is thinking a bit harder about how we might find a way of concretely encouraging more of them to occur more frequently. We've already highlighted two obvious things to do: stop gratuitously driving smart young people away from the field and being on guard against the unscientific influence emanating from the nearby medical community. Is there anything else that should be considered?

I should say at the outset that the basis of the exercise is to consider how a *universal* increase in funds for basic biological research should be spent to the greatest possible effect, without in any way redistributing resources from current programs. Nobody comes away from our thought experiment with less money than they had before.

All too often whenever you ask this sort of question, particularly to a group of academics, you're met with blank looks. In their eyes, the self-evident answer to the problem of "chronic underfunding" (which is indeed a chronic lament) is simply a curt "more money across the board," punctuated by a brazen few stepping up to clarify that, while more resources in general are clearly necessary, their own particular research avenue happens to be the most intrinsically worthy, or the most in need after years of systematic neglect, or the most likely to lead to transformative results, or whatever.

Of course more money in general will surely have an effect, but the vital question is, Is this the **best** way to proceed? Perhaps there are entirely different types of approaches to consider: those representing differences in kind rather than degree, whose potential implementation might result in a significantly more enhanced level of success than just a broad-based funding increase?

Lewis Thomas certainly thought so.

> *"It is time to develop a new group of professional thinkers, perhaps a somewhat larger group than the working scientists, who can create a discipline of scientific criticism. We have had good luck so far in the emergence of a few people ranking as philosophers of science and historians and journalists of science, and I hope more of these will be coming along, but we have not yet seen a Ruskin or a*

*Leavis or an Edmund Wilson. Science needs critics of this sort, but the public at large needs them more urgently.*"[8]

It is truly remarkable how many times Lewis Thomas has penned some telling sociological insight that strongly resonates with something I've independently mused over. There is much to unpack here, from the role of the media to the function of criticism to raising the level of public debate, but the point that immediately galvanized my attention was the possibility that philosophers and historians of science might concretely assist the scientific process itself, both directly (through productive interaction with scientists) and indirectly (by forcing scientists to more rigorously structure any theories they might be inclined to develop).

I've been mulling over this issue for a very long time now. It began when I was a student bouncing back and forth between physics and philosophy, and found myself increasingly bewildered by what a "philosopher of physics" actually was. Was Einstein a "philosopher of physics"? Was Schrödinger? If so, why did present-day philosophers of physics not even try to act like those giants did and propose new scientific ideas through publishing in contemporary physics journals? A common response I'd hear was something like, *Well, there was a time when working physicists were routinely concerned with key philosophical issues but that was long ago; nowadays a yawning sociological divide exists between physicists who develop their theories and philosophers who try to fully understand their implications and put them in their proper overall context* (the wording is inevitably much more abstruse, but it always seemed to boil down to something like that).

This answer has never made the slightest amount of sense to me. Aside altogether from the obvious fact that there have been many deeply influential and thoughtful contemporary physicists with obviously profound philosophical sensitivities (Roger Penrose springs immediately to mind), the very idea that someone who is capable of developing

---

[8] "Humanities and Science" from *Late Night Thoughts on Listening to Mahler's Ninth Symphony*

a theory should then need someone else to appropriately "understand it" or "interpret it" has always struck me as nothing less than the acme of inanity, with a twist of condescension thrown in for good measure.

Of course it was definitely true that attitudes within the sociology of physics ebbed and flowed, as happens in all sociologies; and for a long time many deep conceptual issues in physics were largely ignored under a dominant "shut up and calculate" mindset. But a quick glance at the historical record reveals that the resurgence of profoundly philosophically-oriented insights in physics actually came through physicists, from John Bell to Alain Aspect to David Deutsch and beyond. To such a list one should clearly add Abner Shimony, a renowned philosopher of science who made seminal contributions to many aspects of fundamental physics, but as he also received a second doctorate in physics under Eugene Wigner, there's no reason to revise the claim. And so the question remained: What is philosophy of physics, really, and what is it good for? Is it actually a thing?

Were it not for the fact that I later found myself in the position of building and running a foundational physics institute, I'm sure I would have long forgotten about the whole business. But as it was, it seemed appropriate to try to press things a bit. So I took the bull by the horns, deliberately engaged with as many members of the global philosophy of science community as possible, and even developed a separate research group (even though we didn't officially have research groups) dedicated to "foundations of quantum theory." In the end I think we managed to create a different sort of research culture through the involvement of some very thoughtful and particularly broad-minded people. But they were all physicists. And by the time I left Perimeter Institute 8 years later I was no closer to understanding what sort of uniquely meaningful role philosophers of science could play in theoretical physics than I was before. Insofar as they were contributing something they were acting like physicists; and insofar as they weren't, they didn't look to be contributing much.

But once I started Ideas Roadshow a few years later and became steadily exposed to the biological world, I started to wonder if perhaps my skepticism about the scientific utility of philosophers of science was simply due to having been focused on the wrong science. Because the more I saw of biology, the more I became independently convinced of the necessity of the sort of clarifying "scientific criticism" that Lewis Thomas had so explicitly recommended, with philosophers potentially playing a leading role.

There are many reasons to imagine why philosophers of science might have a much greater impact in assisting biologists than physicists, from the vastly greater scope of biology that naturally calls out for some sort of synoptic treatment, to its relatively underdeveloped theoretical side, to the sheer, overwhelming number of its participants. But one reason that clearly *doesn't* apply, in direct reinforcement of my earlier comments, is the slightest implication that biologists, being somehow naturally mushier and less rigorous than physicists, need more help to straighten out their thoughts.

It is not so much that being forced to listen to "physics imperialists" insinuate how smart they are is highly irritating (which is surely true), but that a clear-eyed, rigorous comparison of the two scientific endeavors could be of significant benefit to both.[9] And who better to conduct a critical, high-level structural comparison of physics and biology than a philosopher of science?

What might that entail? Well, the obvious starting point would be to explicitly contrast the inherent complexity of the biological world with the essentially reductionist approach of physics. In other words, rather than focus on the notion that physics is "more mathematical" than biology (which is undeniably true), with the consequent implication that biology is therefore "easier" (which is undeniably false), spend

---

[9] My focus here is on the possible advantages accruing to biology from such an exercise, but there are doubtless corresponding insights for physicists as well, although it is much less likely that they would listen, of course.

some time concretely examining why things are different in the two fields.

Doing so will quickly make several key points immediately apparent, such as the general effectiveness in physics of distinguishing between fundamental properties (e.g. mass, charge) and "extraneous features" (e.g. friction, air resistance, deviations from spherical symmetry), with the consequent opportunity to regard a vast array of physical systems through the prism of being composed of, to all intents and purposes, the same underlying constituents with the same core properties and thus naturally subjected to the notion of a universal law that is instantiated in a mathematical equation.

Biology, meanwhile, has hitherto largely resisted such an approach owing to the breathtaking levels of complexity involved on a striking number of different levels: from the combinatorics of genetic information, to the complexities of protein structure to the panoply of individual cellular processes, to the mysteriously coordinated processes of millions of different cells as part of different physiological "systems," to the structural interaction of different organs within a body, to the near-unimaginable variety of species of different types of "bodies," to the feedback mechanisms of ecosystems of zillions of species, to the interplay of huge numbers of different ecosystems in the biosphere and much more besides.

It is not just that biology can be phenomenally, almost inconceivably complicated. It's that its very complexity *itself* is hellishly complicated. All of which make it distinctly problematic, if not at times downright impossible, to try to distinguish between "fundamental" and "extraneous" as a physicist might, with all the corresponding frustration of being able to meaningfully address the most basic sort of question to kick-start the knowledge process like, "What is a gene?" or "What is a species?" let alone something like, "Why are all the proteins found in the human body made up of only 4% of the amino acids found in nature?"

And yet there are revealing crossovers between the two. There are many instances in physics, such as the famous "butterfly effect" in non-linear systems, when the causal impact of instabilities in your framework are maddeningly unpredictable—when it is, to put it mildly, highly non-trivial if not impossible to be able to successfully differentiate between notions of "fundamental" and "extraneous." There are also, just as revealingly, a great many examples in physics of different phenomena, or types of phenomena, that manifest themselves at very different levels, with all the inherent challenges of clearly delineating where the dividing line between such levels actually is and what could conceivably be responsible for it

Meanwhile, there are occasions in biology, such as the "reading of the genetic code," when a similar sort of physics-esque reductionist approach yields manifold dividends, with "fundamental" processes being procured by specific genes and "diseases" logically viewed as the inhibition of the production of the appropriate protein due to the mutation of the corresponding gene. Given the manifold complexities of the biological world, such analogies often break down quite quickly, with genes being a long conceptual distance away from the "point particles" of physics, but getting a better understanding of where, exactly, such breakdowns occur (and thus why) would in itself, I'm certain, be very useful. And once again, that's precisely the sort of activity that philosophers of science are ideally qualified to engage in.

In short, I can't help but think that if you were somehow able to take all the philosophers of physics active today and direct them to contrast their deep understanding of physics with that of contemporary biology it would be of considerable objective benefit to both the philosophers and the biologists, and no significant loss to physics (the physicists, I'm sure, wouldn't even notice that they were gone).[10]

---

[10] The possibility of applying biological insights to physics has, as you might imagine, been significantly less remarked upon than extending physics-based approaches to biology, but one intriguing example I know of is Lee Smolin's theory of "Cosmological Natural Selection" as outlined in his book, *Life of the Cosmos*.

One concrete aspect of the sort of "scientific criticism" that Lewis Thomas was calling for, then, involves a rigorous comparison of physics and biology. What might some others be?

Personally, I can think of three more particularly helpful types of criticism within biology itself.

The first involves making a dedicated effort to focus on important issues that would otherwise go unnoticed. By this I mean two things:

> 1. Renewing interest in specific, unexplained phenomena that have, in the course of time, somehow been swept under the scientific rug. Lewis Thomas, as will surely not surprise you by now, paid particularly vigorous attention to this sort of thing, regularly writing about a wide range of phenomena—from animal communication to warts to the effects of hypnosis on the immune system to canine olfactory detection (COVID-19 sniffing dogs anyone?)—that intriguingly eluded our understanding and correspondingly opened up a cascade of fascinating questions that largely hadn't been followed up on.

> 2. Explicitly highlighting potentially transformative conceptual ideas that would otherwise lie unappreciated. What I have in mind here is the much-ballyhooed notion of "interdisciplinarity," the go-to word of academic administrators the world over whenever they want to justify any course of action. But despite their best efforts, the concept still has—just—some remnants of semantic content associated with it, particularly so in research domains that are so conspicuously broad that it is quite conceivable that a core conceptual advance in one subdomain hasn't yet had time to filter down to another.

An example will help here, I think. During my recent conversation with Miguel Nicolelis, he mentioned a specific epidemiological hypothesis he was developing about a relationship between infection rates of different RNA viruses (Dengue, influenza and COVID-19) that was motivated by his conviction that the brain and the immune system had fundamental structural similarities in terms of the way in which they processed information.

The key idea is that, just as the brain and the central nervous system actively develop a representation of the outside world that is constantly refined through incoming sense data, the immune system might do something similar, creating its own representation of "immunological reality" that is subsequently adjusted in the light of immunological evidence.

This is, I think, a very intriguing idea, which, if true, could well have a transformative impact on our fundamental understanding of basic immunological processes. Of course, it might not: it might be poorly defined, or boil down to something we already currently believe, or be just plain wrong. But given the enormously broad landscape of what we mean by "biology," it is all too likely that when a world-leading neuroscientist says, "*Here's this particular epidemiological hypothesis that I've developed based upon applying a core conceptual insight about how the brain operates to immunological systems,*" very few in the world of immunology or epidemiology will pay the slightest attention to him, disdainfully responding, if at all, "*Stick to your neuroscience.*" Or perhaps the only thing they'll focus on is the specific hypothesis in question about RNA viruses—which could turn out to be, in itself, poorly constructed or just plain wrong—and whose significance pales in comparison to its guiding conceptual insight, which might still be right.

That there is an important role critical outsiders can play in drawing increased attention to insights that might otherwise go overlooked is not, of course, to declare that biologists are particularly conservative or closed-minded or what have you. They are not (given proper attention to the word "particularly"). But it is an exceptionally large scientific community and everyone is busy. Moreover, this is precisely the sort of thing that philosophers of science, with their broad analytical training, are extremely well-suited to.

A third very valuable critical function that they are particularly well-suited to is the ability to point out muddled thinking. Once more it might be worth stressing that I hardly believe that biologists are the only types of scientists who are prone to regularly making elementary philosophical transgressions,[11] but it cannot be denied that the biological world is routinely littered with them, from the constant conflation of statistical correlation with causation to the longstanding denial of the evolutionary importance of sleep, despite its flagrant all-pervasiveness throughout the biological world.[12]

And then there is the all-too-frequent lack of sufficiently thinking things through in advance of an experiment. A particularly prominent example of this was revealed to me by Stephen Scherer during our first Ideas Roadshow conversation[13] when he described how, since the Human Genome Project was explicitly designed to throw away any deviations in donor DNA from the "common linear sequence," the entire (enormously expensive) exercise was logically incapable of detecting what Stephen and his colleagues discovered only a few years later: that a dramatically larger proportion of genes than we had long believed can participate in the evolutionary process through varying their so-called copy number.

But the most consistent advertisement for the need for critical philosophical thinking in biology occurs whenever the highly distorting combination of teleological tendencies and anthropomorphization

---

[11] For one particularly egregious example from the world of physics, see Paul Steinhardt's terse description of the profound philosophical incoherence of many proponents of inflationary cosmology, in chapter 5 of *Inflated Expectations: A Cosmological Tale–A Conversation with Paul Steinhardt*.

[12] Famously summed up by pioneering sleep scientist Allan Rechtschaffen's curiously necessary remark: "*If sleep does not serve an absolutely vital function, then it is the biggest mistake in evolutionary history."*

[13] *Our Human Variability–A Conversation with Stephen Scherer*

begin to creep into evolutionary discourse—which is unfortunately very often indeed.

To take one particularly timely example, think of how often these days you've heard talk of "the evolutionary strategy" of the SARS-CoV-2 virus, or invocations of a "cat and mouse" game between humans and the virus, with the virus desperately trying to evade our souped-up defense mechanisms by evolving into something different. This might sound like simply a convenient, shorthand way of describing what's going on in order to make it broadly accessible, but such false representations have a well-demonstrated tendency to lead us down a perilous garden path.

Because if you really believe that the virus is "implementing a strategy," it follows that any subsequent mutation will necessarily be less dangerous to our health than the one before, because, after all, it is "in the virus' best interest" that we stay alive as long as possible so that we can, in turn, successfully pass copies of it on to others (who will do likewise).

But the truth is that the virus doesn't think that way, because the virus doesn't think. At all. The virus just *is*.[14] And mutations of the virus, so far as we can tell, just happen. Of course once they do happen, then it's not unreasonable to judge which ones are going to be more "successful" (from the virus' perspective) than others, just as it's perfectly reasonable to conclude that if both humans and some form of the SARS-CoV-2 virus are going to be around in 500 years then that form of the SARS-CoV-2 virus will be relatively benign to us, but that's a completely different sort of thing from saying that the virus is now "implementing its strategy." It has no strategy. And so there is no reason to believe that the next mutation tomorrow will necessarily

---

[14] I am generally opposed to human-centric approaches to the biological world that dismiss the ratiocination abilities of other creatures, and am quite convinced that my dog has more intellectual perspicacity than most people, but I draw the line at viruses.

be inherently "more benign" to us than today's.[15] Our hope, rather, is that our collective immune systems have been sufficiently prepared to respond effectively to whatever, within reasonable limits, happens to come our way.

The perceptive reader will have noticed that this last example represents a subtle drift in the target of our putative "scientific criticism" from the scientific community to the general public, thereby underscoring Thomas' concluding comment that, "*Science needs critics of this sort, but the public at large needs them more urgently.*" It is not, of course, that biologists never confuse evolution with teleology (if only), but by far the greater danger in such misunderstanding lies with the general public, particularly during a large-scale health crisis.

Which brings me to our last general category of how a well-constructed system of "scientific criticism" might be best poised to simultaneously assist biology and society at large. To review, so far I've mentioned comparing the structural difference between physics and biology, focusing people's attention on outstanding biological mysteries and innovative, interdisciplinary ideas that would otherwise go unrecognized, and diligently providing philosophical oversight to identify and promptly rectify any muddled thinking that has arisen.

The fourth category is a steadfast examination and appraisal of our present biological moment and concomitant future potential, consistently seeking out a "big picture perspective" in an attempt to distinguish the transformative from the incremental. This sort of thing is necessarily speculative, but no less important because of that.

It also provides a concrete mechanism for expanding the domain of "scientific criticism" well beyond philosophy of science. Science journalists, in particular, are likely to retort that placing contemporary

---

[15] Some clever virologist may well one day come up with a framework that demonstrates that there is, in fact, some sort of internal structural relationship in viral-host mechanics between, say, transmissibility and toxicity—what do I know?—but that is, of course, quite beside the point being made here.

scientific activity in its proper perspective while speculating on its future impact is, in fact, their day job.

It's difficult to argue with such a statement, largely because it's hard to know with any degree of certainty what, exactly, the day job of a science journalist is supposed to be anyway, but it's certainly true that the best sorts of science journalists are indeed strongly oriented in precisely this direction. But aside from the candid observation that there simply aren't very many of those around, is the more telling concern that attempts to assess when we are genuinely living through "revolutionary moments"—always difficult—are made all the more complicated still by a sensationalizing media perpetually bent on convincing us of the transformative impact of every item they are reporting on, resulting in a continually overhyped culture that a journalist friend of mine once pithily characterized as "black holes coming out of your nose."

Legitimately trying to sort out the scientific wheat from the chaff, on the other hand, is much harder. It requires a good deal of knowledge, historical context, investigative ability and reflection. But it is very much worth it, because if done right there is scope to make a highly valuable contribution to both public and scientific understanding.

One obvious recent development that is clearly in the process of transforming biology is the rapidly expanding role of computer simulations and mathematical modeling, not only in the traditional terms of hardware and software (drastic increases in processing power and an exploding array of machine-learning algorithms), but also through the enormous influx of computer scientists and modelers into the field. There is clearly huge promise there. But there is also a correspondingly great need to engage in much careful critical work to do our best to ensure that we use the tools and techniques to their full potential and not fall into the sorts of knee-jerk, unreflective paeans to "Big Data" as has been done in the past, blithely assuming that the biggest calculator will necessarily lead to the biggest insight. It will not.

Another great example of a potentially revolutionary change in biology is represented by the recent mRNA vaccine. Yet another curious aspect of a global pandemic—well, this one, anyway—is that it somehow leads to far greater numbers of people unceasingly holding forth on "the implications of mRNA vaccines" than those who have any real understanding of what mRNA actually is. This state of affairs naturally makes it particularly difficult to get any real sense of what is going on. Are we living in a historically significant moment? If so, why, exactly? What does it mean?

Here's Stephen Scherer's analysis of what makes this "mRNA moment" so special:

> *"You're building on information that you're introducing into the system or the cells or the organs—whatever it may be—to harness the existing biology to modulate some process. In this case it's the immune response to fight off the virus. The conceptual leap forward is that you can now deliver this information stably into the cells, so now everyone's eyes are wide open: 'Well, if we can do this for a piece of this virus, maybe we can do it for some of the genes that are missing in the 6000 rare diseases and even think about delivering it to organs like the brain, which were previously seen as inaccessible?'"*

One simple paragraph and it's all there: no distracting jargon-laden details of the subtleties of lipid nanoparticles or ribosomes or toll-like receptors, however necessary they obviously are to understanding the operational mechanics of the mRNA vaccine. What makes this a potentially transformative moment is our newfound ability to directly transmit information to our cells so as to engage our natural cellular mechanisms in the production of what we need (or inhibit production of what we don't want).

That's the sort of message that desperately needs to be neatly packaged and widely reiterated time and again to everyone—even otherwise distracted scientists, who might suddenly sit up and say to themselves, "*Hang on a minute, maybe that means I could do my research in a slightly different way...*"

In addition to science journalists, this final category of "scientific criticism" also strongly encourages historians of science to actively participate, not least because assessing "historical moments" properly involves comparing and contrasting the present with the past.

But there are several other reasons too for scientists to pay careful attention to what historians of science have to say. As Lorraine Daston reflected:

> "*Scientists are living in a situation of extraordinary uncertainty and they don't know how the story is going to end—that is their actual daily reality. And yet all the history that is told to them in their textbooks and also by way of anecdote is teleological:* '**At first we knew nothing, and then there was this result and that result and finally light dawned, it crystallized into the answer, which has taken us to where we are now.**
>
> "*That way of narrating the history is so incongruous with one's lived experience that one could understand why the scientists themselves tend to minimize it in their own researches. Moreover, in this period of extraordinary acceleration of scientific results and corresponding specialization, they have often lost the overview of,* **Why are we studying the things we are studying now? What would be the alternatives?**
>
> "*Uprooting the narrative of teleology and giving a more panoramic view of both the justification of and possible alternatives to present research activities are two ways how the history of science could be of use to scientists.*"

And then there's the frequently overlooked point that some long-dead scientists might actually have something particularly valuable to contribute to our current understanding. Generally speaking, of course, science is rightly seen as a steady accumulation of methodically-acquired knowledge, continually refined. But the conclusion that some implicitly leap to—*Therefore the past has nothing to teach us and any significant advancement of our knowledge is necessarily fully incorporated in current thinking so all we need to do is read the most recent papers*—is naive at best.

Sometimes great ideas get overlooked. Sometimes we go down the wrong path. And sometimes we find that people who lived a century or two ago developed particularly keen insights on some of the very same problems that we're currently struggling with.

One example that always comes to mind in this regard is Hermann von Helmholtz, whose numerous seminal insights have spontaneously arisen in more Ideas Roadshow conversations than I can remember. The idea that someone so profoundly perceptive has nothing more to teach us merely because he had the misfortune to have died 128 years ago has long struck me as nothing less than absurd.

Helmholtz, as it happens, was a physicist. And a biologist. And a philosopher of science. We owe it to ourselves to pull out all the stops to find and support as many future Helmholtzes as we can, as quickly as possible.

## 10. Conclusion

> *"These ought to be the best of times for the human mind, but it is not so. I cannot begin to guess at all the causes of our cultural sadness, not even the most important ones, but I can think of one thing that is wrong with us and eats away at us: we do not know enough about ourselves."*[1]

But doing biology better is not enough. As mentioned in the first chapter, when I began my *Pandemic Perspectives* journey, that was all I thought I'd be focusing on. Then I thought it was going to be about assessing our governance structures, or information dissemination mechanisms, or research culture, or level of scientific literacy, or capabilities of critical thinking, or the relationship between our stated values with how we actually act during a crisis. The goal, you may recall, was to "harness the pandemic"—capitalizing on this unique moment in time to generate valuable insights on a spectrum of societal issues that might otherwise remain obscured, so that when everything is over, when we "return to normal," we can at least be in a position of having learned something from the whole miserable affair.

But that, too, I now know, is the wrong way to look at it. Because the pandemic isn't simply, as I cavalierly announced in the film's introduction, "a brutally-jolting worldwide timeout." It turns out that it is a harbinger, a message, a concrete demonstration that we are well and truly in a "new normal" that we had better start coming to terms with before it is too late.

---

[1] "Medical Lessons from History" in *The Medusa and the Snail*

I am not the sort of person to typically use such apocalyptic-sounding language, which I've long believed can be decidedly counterproductive. As everyone knows, the environmental movement has long had an unfortunate penchant for screaming about imminent global destruction, often buttressed by Hollywood executives salivating at the chance to combine high-grossing disaster films with sanctimonious self-importance (e.g. *The Day After Tomorrow*) as they zoom off in their block-long limos to attend another self-congratulatory award ceremony.

It all seemed more designed to irritate people than generate any substantively different behavior—which is, on the whole, pretty well what happened. "Environmental movements" did slowly gain a sort of momentum, but were all-too-typically slotted into the all-encompassing political spectrum as being firmly on "the left"—as if hunters and golfers and bankers were somehow wholly indifferent to the beauty of the natural world or the importance of healthy ecosystems and clean air—with self-proclaimed "progressives" doing their utmost to ensure that it stayed there by sanctimoniously lining up behind a messianic finger-wagging high-school dropout.

Wrong, wrong, wrong. Or better still, to invoke the legendary Wolfgang Pauli yet again: "Not even wrong."[2]

Because it is not just that this particular specter of environmental degradation transcends any reasonable difference in public policy choices that any coherent definition of "political divide" logically entails. It's that virtually **all** of our pressing problems these days transcend our current mechanisms for dealing with them.

**This** is what the pandemic so stunningly reveals; and it does so precisely because it is *not* (at least not directly) an environmental issue. Like most people, I used to look at "environmental issues" as some sort of collective exception to the general order of things. Most problems could

---

[2] I told you I was going to do this; it is really quite unavoidable.

be dealt with locally or nationally, I figured, but "environmental things" like climate change or species extinction clearly needed a different sort of approach—some sort of truly "global governance" solution perhaps, with the primary challenge being how to convince national governments to collectively yield sovereignty to any international body with the power to implement meaningful change.

But the pandemic put paid to that line of thinking: here was an entirely different type of serious problem that we also clearly cannot deal with under our present structure. It's not because we are necessarily unwilling or incompetent, or that our "leaders" are lousy, or that we've made poor decisions, or that we don't have the right technology—some of that may be the case or none of it—it's because we simply don't have the right tools. You can't write a novel with a violin; and it doesn't make the slightest difference if you happen to have a Stradivarius. It's not the right tool for the job.

I'm sure you're getting awfully tired of this by now, but I'm compelled to report that Lewis Thomas tried very hard to alert us to this too.

I've mentioned on repeated occasions my amazement at how virtually every step I took on this *Pandemic Perspectives* journey revealed that Lewis Thomas had been there years before me, writing penetratingly about its promise or perils. But the one Thomasian theme I was certain I could skip over, the few essays that I was convinced were *not* going to be relevant to my pandemic peregrination, were those desperately highlighting the utter madness of our inexplicable determination to flirt with the prospect of global thermonuclear war. Written as they were in the early 1980s, they were, I assured myself, clearly a relic of a bygone era—most understandably motivated, of course, given the circumstances, but now mercifully irrelevant.

But no. And it's not just because I write these words as Vladimir Putin explicitly threatens using nuclear weapons as part of his delusional ravings linked to the horrifying invasion of Ukraine (although that can hardly be ignored), but more generally because current global political crises such as this vividly represent yet another example still—together with the pandemic and numerous deeply troubling environmental concerns—of the inherently global nature of our current problems that simply cannot be solved by our current national political structures.

Like it or not, as Fedya Kondrashov aptly described it earlier, "*We are truly, really, all in the same boat.*" And if we don't collectively wake up to that reality we are all in very serious trouble indeed. It almost doesn't matter which crisis we somehow manage to avoid by a fortuitous fluke (like Mikhael Gorbachev coming to power in the mid-1980s)—which array of bullets we manage to dodge by a happy concatenation of circumstances—sooner or later our luck is bound to run out. Counting on fate to solve your existential threats is a remarkably poor strategy.

And put in this context it starts becoming increasingly clear that we actually have been pretty lucky so far, because the ground has been shifting for the better part of a century now. The "Cold War" was not a "thing that we got over" any more than climate change became "real" when the IPCC was formed in 1988.

It wasn't always this way, of course. If you lived in classical Athens or precolonial Australia or China during the Ming Dynasty, then your appropriate "political domain" was obviously not a global one. You might well find yourself attacked by foreign invaders to the point where you faced existential threats, but they were local existential threats—i.e. threats to you and not the planet as a whole—and thus naturally entailed local solutions that some were able to meet and others were not. This might not make much difference to you if your group was the one facing extinction, but it makes a big difference from a planetary perspective.

And when you look closely, you see that, in fact, matters have been "necessarily global" for quite some time now; it's just taken most of us much longer to recognize it than it should have. The proper way to look at things is not that Lewis Thomas lived "way back in the Cold War era," it's simply that he lived a little bit earlier than we did in the "necessarily global era"; and being considerably more astute than most of his fellow travelers, he noticed it much quicker. In fact, he noticed it roughly a half century or so before I did, without needing to be pushed into it by a global pandemic. It's never pleasant to be confronted with your own shortcomings, but there it is: make a film about a pandemic and discover your own obliviousness. Learning is learning.

The main question now, however, is how to move forwards. Given that we find ourselves firmly ensconced in the "necessarily global" era with only flagrantly locally-oriented political structures, there seem to me only two possible solutions: "upscale" existing political structures to a suitably international level or somehow transform them so that they can meaningfully address inherently global concerns.

The first approach has already been tried, most notably with the creation of The United Nations System, International Criminal Court and all of that. And while there have surely been a number of isolated success stories, and it's demonstrably true that a world with the UN is incomparably superior to one without one, it seems frankly impossible to imagine creating any possible "scaled up" version of national politics with a "President of the World" with a clear mandate to safeguard the health and welfare of all earthlings equally.

You don't have to be confronted with extreme examples of brutal nationalist warmongers like Vladimir Putin to appreciate the obvious point that nobody currently holding any significant degree of political power would be willing to cede sovereignty over their domain to some third party.

Equally relevantly, it is almost as difficult to imagine that the citizens themselves, if somehow given a choice, would do so under current circumstances. A mere glance at the European Union's (non-)response to the pandemic—where 27 wealthy, culturally-related members of a regional collective were comprehensively incapable of coordinating the most basic emergency responses to an urgent health threat—should convince anyone that "global governance" as commonly envisioned is about as likely to happen as 100 monkeys banging out 100 different plays of Sophocles in one go.[3]

Which brings us to option two: transforming politics somehow to enable us to successfully address our current and future global challenges.

I'll consider later to what extent what I'm about to suggest can be regarded as the slightest bit "realistic," but for the moment it's worth admitting that I am hardly suffused with positive feelings about the whole business. But when facing an existential threat to which the only escape you can envision involves betting the house on 100 spontaneously Sophoclean monkeys, it behooves you to go back to the drawing board and come up with an alternative, however unlikely.

So here goes.

By "transforming politics" what I have in mind is not some form of more efficient governance framework, which, when scaled globally as it logically needs to be, brings us squarely back to the aforementioned simian playwright probabilities. No, that is both hopeless and—even more significantly—squarely beside the point, as America's current state of political dysfunctionality amply attests to. This is not, by any objective measure, the fault of their Constitution, which most observers both inside and outside the country have long concluded is quite a good one. So rolling up our sleeves and trying to somehow come up with a better one still, even assuming that it could conceivably be implemented—which it obviously couldn't—is nothing less than a waste of time of monumental proportions, roughly akin to trying to jump to the moon in order to cure your toothache: you can't do it; and even if you somehow could it wouldn't actually help the situation in the slightest.

---

[3] Which naturally includes, for those of you who are paying attention to such things, the 93 or so that are currently lost to us.

What I'm proposing instead is to go right back to first principles and spend some time investigating what the point of what is commonly understood as "politics" is in the first place, to investigate if there is room to somehow refocus there, at least with some significant portion of the population. And to help me along, I'm going to invoke the assistance of my partner-in-arms John Dunn, citing some of his trenchant comments from our recent podcast conversation.

First, a recapitulation of the challenge before us:

> *"We are in ever-deepening trouble as a species; and there's no hope at all of us getting out of that trouble unless more of us come to recognize that and care about it."*

Note that the implied solution, or road to a solution, isn't the slightest bit structural. He's not saying, *"There's no hope at all of us getting out of that trouble unless we do away with the Electoral College"* or *"...unless we institute proportional representation"* or *"...unless we transform the Security Council"* or even *"...unless we throw out leader X and replace him with leader Y"* or anything like that. Instead the way forward straightforwardly requires sufficient numbers of people to be upset by the current situation and wish to do something about it.

So that's the first point: politics is primarily a vehicle for changing things in our social world that we are worried about. The reason why the steadily diminishing use of apostrophes in the English language has not become "a political issue" in any anglophone country that I know of is not because political issues can never be linguistically-oriented or that apostrophes are inherently "politically neutral," but simply because nobody gives a damn about it.[4]

Which brings up the next pivotal question: Who is most likely to be concerned about the status quo and why?

---

[4] Other than me.

# Conclusion

I've spent a lot of time puzzling over this lately, because to my mind it is structurally linked to the most profoundly perplexing question imaginable: *Why don't enough people sufficiently care about the way things are going so that we can collectively engage in finding a way to develop meaningful solutions to our very serious problems?*

Rather than trying to address this question head-on, which takes us into all sorts of depressing, detailed discussions on the woeful state of public education or the corporatization of the media or whatever, let's instead recognize that this is actually a variant of the question: *Why do so many people feel compelled to take politics as it is presently constituted so seriously?*

Because they clearly do. Whether it's becoming teary-eyed at the inauguration of the first African-American president or vigorously decrying the transparently mind-controlling ambitions of the European Union or patriotically attacking "running dogs of capitalism" or donning red acronymed caps to manifest your allegiance to a power-crazed buffoon, people all around the world evidently care enormously about this sort of thing. Somehow, inexplicably, a great many human beings are convinced that these sorts of things matter enormously to their daily lives.

But they actually don't.

So, what to do? Well, one common approach is to try to tell people that their particular beliefs associated with this overall framework are wrong: that it is right to feel teary-eyed at the inauguration of the first African-American president, say, but it is wrong to passionately roar your approval at the words of the power-crazed buffoon (or vice-versa).

This is, to put it mildly, very unlikely to work.[5]

What needs to be done, I think, is not to try to convince people that their specific allegiances under the current structure are wrong, but

---

[5] I speak from some experience here.

rather that the entire *structure* is wrong—indeed, dangerously so: that none of the specific alternatives on offer under the current structure actually care about you or your long-term welfare; and, consequently, whatever they say or do is very unlikely to be of direct benefit to your everyday life. And that we can do things better.

At this point two obvious objections will doubtless be hurled my way.

The first is to say that, while such criticisms undoubtedly apply to non-democratic types of government, they are fundamentally misplaced when describing democracies, which are, tautologically, representations of the people's will. And any system that produces a result that is a faithful representation of what people actually believe is necessarily aligned with their interests, otherwise you are forced to conclude that people don't generally want what is in their interests, which is absurd.

There is a fairly straightforward four-fold reply to this one:

> 1. Unenthusiastically marking a ballot every few years to enable the least repugnant person to make decisions on my behalf is a very long way indeed from an expression of how I would like my life to improve.

> 2. There is a constantly-reinforced structural mechanism to ensure that I will always be presented with nothing other than generally repugnant options, since the only way someone can get on the ballot in the first place is through a highly concentrated decades-long effort for personal power, which necessarily precludes anyone who is not inherently power-hungry from the game (and don't get me started on the self-congratulatory trope of "a long, distinguished career of public service" that we are forced to swallow on a disturbingly regular basis).

> 3. Even if it could be reasonably maintained that current democratic systems are faithful representations of what people

actually want (which it can't—see above), there is a big difference between someone's short-term desires and her long-term interests; and the very mechanisms of our current democratic practices necessarily favor the former at the expense of the latter, with a consequent tendency to downplay or even downright deny any long-term threats. And given that most of the threats we are concerned about here are long-term, this is particularly disastrous.

4. To all of this should be added the clarifying remark that just because a system is better than existing alternatives doesn't mean that it is in any way good. That I generally prefer current democratic structures to their alternatives—which I most certainly do; I live in France, after all—is hardly an endorsement of their efficacy in and of itself, but only in their *relative* efficacy; which, given our situation, is not saying very much.

So much for the first objection.

The second one, however, is considerably more concerning:

*Let's say you're right—that the core problem is that there are millions (billions?) of people out there who are incorrectly convinced that politics as currently constructed actually represents their true interests. How on earth can this possibly be changed?*

At this point I feel obliged to reiterate my earlier comment that the goal here is to come up with a solution that is more likely than a century of suddenly Sophoclean monkeys, which is a very far cry indeed from manifesting an unbridled sense of optimism. I am not, as you have surely gathered by now, particularly optimistic about things. But still.

It may well be, as Darrin McMahon speculated when grappling with why the devastation of the pandemic seemed to have such a mysteriously minimal impact on changing people's perspective, that things first have to get a whole lot worse before they get any better.

> *"Despite the terrible social cost of this pandemic, it may be that it doesn't cut deep enough to really prompt the kind of change that major tragedies in the past have. If you think about the aftermath of the Second World War with all the carnage and all the destruction and all the diseases that followed, human beings were really ready for significant change in all kinds of ways. And I fear that, despite the great tragedy of this pandemic and all the loss in human life, that it may not be bad enough to urge us to make the kind of changes that we need to make in order to live in a better world."*

The vital silver lining behind these comments is the indisputable fact that, whatever truly horrific events were required to force us to get to that point, there are at least one or two legitimate historical precedents of having collectively decided to change our behavior so as to live in a better world.

If there is any hope at all, I'm convinced, it has to come from the young. Not only because the older generations are both far too set in their ways and far too personally invested in the status quo, and not only because revolutions are a particularly fun thing to be engaged in when you've got lots of time and energy and a strong desire to rebel against those who've long been telling you what to do, but most importantly because young people today are clearly going to be directly affected by the sorts of global problems we've been discussing.

In all likelihood nobody over the age of 50 is going to have to directly worry about the sorts of things I've been discussing here (always assuming we don't blow up the world tomorrow). But if you're 15, or 25, or even 35, it's an entirely different story: your opportunity to live a good, flourishing life is very much under threat.

Ironic though it most certainly is, it seems that it's come to this: putting all of my hopes in the sort of "enlightened self-interest" arguments so near and dear to those dreaded, oft-pilloried microeconomists. Well, every dog has its day.

When I asked John Dunn, towards the end of our podcast conversation, what he would say to a young person today to assuage her that the future wasn't hopeless, he had this to say.

> *"Well, I wouldn't be able to tell her that it's not hopeless, because that would be a lie—I'm not convinced that it isn't. I would talk to her in a different way, I suppose. I would say: 'You should read The Death of Ivan Ilyich.' You want to think of your life in terms of how it's going to feel to you as it ends. And what is going to be most important at that point is what you feel about the life you have lived in terms of what you truly believe to be of value."*

This duly sent me scurrying back to reread Tolstoy's "The Death of Ivan Ilyich," a novella I only very dimly remembered. It turns out to be an astonishingly moving portrayal of a dying man who has "always done the right thing" who ultimately realizes that he has wasted his life by mindlessly following societal mores rather than following his inner beliefs and values. It could not be more apt to our story. Have I mentioned that I am very fond of John Dunn?

It is also particularly apt that, at a time when pundits are imperiously bombarding us with their "realpolitik" analysis of the "intellectual coherence" of Vladimir Putin's psychotic determination to re-impose "Russian domination" by de facto "re-establishing the Soviet Union," John's invocation of Tolstoy's timeless insights is a tangible example of genuine "Russian domination" on a global scale that necessarily has nothing to do with being Russian at all. For that's what all this business about "the human condition" actually means: being human.[6]

---

[6] Those who can't help but think in the usual "realpolitik" way—which is almost everyone over the age of 15—might want to bear in mind Michael Berry's comments on the United States' recent gratuitous alienation of China

My message, then, to young people is simply this:

Everything you see around you is wrong: newspaper editorials, media analysis, what your parents tell you, "politics," "international relations," the whole shebang. **None** of it will help you in the slightest—indeed, it will most assuredly *hurt* you. In short: following in our footsteps, doing "the right thing" according to "our current world-view" is nothing less than a one-way ticket to Ivan Ilyich-like perdition.

In particular, please pay no attention whatsoever to the huge numbers of people around you who will unhesitatingly inform you that such a revolution isn't possible, that you are being "ridiculously unrealistic." I have no doubt that the very same sorts of comments were leveled at the young people on Easter Island hundreds of years ago who were quite reasonably pointing out:

*"You know, if we keep destroying our habitat to erect all of these moai, we're going to have pretty lousy lives very soon."*

*"Ah young people today!"* I can imagine the smug reply. *"So unrealistic."*

So please, ignore them all: make a revolution. Change the world. Change *your* world. We had our chance, and we screwed it up thoroughly. Now it's your turn to figure out a better way of collective action, of being political.

Just remember this: Politics, as Alex Quintanilha so penetratingly expressed it, doesn't have the luxury of time. And neither do you.

And while you're at it, you might want to consider doing some biology too. There's a lot of cool stuff out there.

---

and contemplate to what extent Mr. Putin's expansionist tendencies might have been better checked had US-Chinese relations not been so needlessly poisoned; but of course, I'm urging people to forego that entire creaky and counterproductive framework.

# Pandemic Perspectives Participants

1. Elizabeth Anderson, University of Michigan
2. Ann-Sophie Barwich, Indiana University Bloomington
3. Roy Baumeister, University of Queensland
4. Michael Berry, UCLA
5. Christopher Celenza, Johns Hopkins University
6. Patricia Churchland, UC San Diego
7. Lorraine Daston, Max Planck Institute for the History of Science
8. John Dunn, University of Cambridge
9. John Dupré, University of Exeter
10. Charles Foster, University of Oxford
11. Richard Frank, Brookings Institution and Harvard University
12. Michael Frazer, University of East Anglia
13. Michael Gordin, Princeton University
14. Joanna Haigh, Imperial College London
15. Brian Hie, Stanford University
16. Andrew Hoffman, University of Michigan
17. Rush Holt, Special Director's Visitor, Institute for Advanced Study
18. Martin Jay, UC Berkeley
19. Paul Kahn, Yale University
20. Philip Kitcher, Columbia University
21. Fyodor Kondrashov, Institute of Science and Technology Vienna
22. Stephen Kosslyn, Active Learning Sciences Inc.
23. Darrin McMahon, Dartmouth College
24. Samuel Moyn, Yale University
25. Miguel Nicolelis, Duke University
26. Caroline Paunov, OECD
27. Alexandre Quintanilha, Member of Portuguese Parliament
28. Teofilo Ruiz, UCLA
29. Stephen Scherer, Toronto Hospital for Sick Children
30. John Tregoning, Imperial College London
31. Gavin Yamey, Duke University
32. Yong Zhao, University of Kansas & Melbourne Grad. School of Education

Visit www.ideasroadshow.com for details about the film and podcasts.

www.ingramcontent.com/pod-product-compliance
Lightning Source LLC
Chambersburg PA
CBHW020255030426
42336CB00010B/774